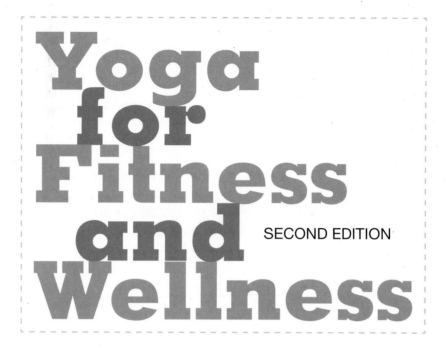

Yoga for Fitness and Wellness

SECOND EDITION

Ravi Dykema

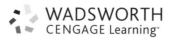

WADSWORTH
CENGAGE Learning

Australia • Brazil • Japan • Korea • Mexico • Singapore • Spain • United Kingdom • United States

WADSWORTH
CENGAGE Learning

Yoga for Fitness and Wellness, Second Edition
Ravi Dykema

Publisher/Executive Editor: Yolanda Cossio

Print Buyer: Judy Inuoye

Right Acquisition Director: Bob Kauser

Permissions Editors: Dean Dauphinais
    (Text & Image)

Production Manager: Matt Ballantyne

Acquisitions Editor: Laura Pople

Assistant Editor: Samantha Arvin

Developmental Editor: Liana Monari Sarkisian

Editorial Assistant/Associate: Kristina Chiapella

Technology Project Manager: Miriam Meyers

Marketing Manager: Laura McGinn

Marketing Assistant/Associate: Elizabeth Wong

Art Director: John Walker

Content Project Management: PreMediaGlobal

Manufacturing Manager: Marcia Locke

Cover Design: Betsy Bush

Cover Images: Masterfile

For product information and technology assistance, contact us at
Cengage Learning Customer & Sales Support, 1-800-354-9706.

For permission to use material from this text or product,
submit all requests online at **cengage.com/permissions**
Further permissions questions can be emailed to
permissionrequest@cengage.com

Library of Congress Control Number: 2010935919

ISBN-13: 978-0-8400-4811-0

ISBN-10: 0-8400-4811-4

Wadsworth
10 Davis Drive
Belmont, CA 94002-3098
USA

Cengage Learning is a leading provider of customized learning solutions with office locations around the globe, including Singapore, the United Kingdom, Australia, Mexico, Brazil, and Japan. Locate your local office at:
international.cengage.com/region

Cengage Learning products are represented in Canada by Nelson Education, Ltd.

For your course and learning solutions, visit **www.cengage.com**

Purchase any of our products at your local college store or at our preferred online store **www.cengagebrain.com**

Printed in the United States of America
2 3 4 5 6 7 14 13 12 11

Contents

Preface

This book is mostly about you—your body and its sensations, your mind and thoughts, your feelings and aspirations. Yoga is the tool we will be using to help you explore these aspects of yourself. Not only does Yoga help you explore yourself, but it can also help you to become healthier, to feel less beaten down by stress, to feel more alert and focused, to sleep better, to gain muscle tone and flexibility, and to feel more alive and energized. When you walk out of a Yoga class, the sky can seem bluer, the sun warmer on your hair, the breeze fresher on your cheek, and your step lighter. You may even feel a gladness and fullness in your heart that just *is,* that doesn't seem to be a response to anything that's happening, such as getting an *A* on a test or thoughts of an upcoming trip. When you feel such fullness you may notice that your attention is on your immediate experience—your sensations, your vision, your hearing—and you may notice that your mental chatter is quieter than usual. That is the goal of most traditional Yoga: to quiet your mind so your present experience becomes more vivid.[1] To achieve this goal, Hatha Yoga uses movement and breathing exercises, combined with concentration. The less physically oriented Yoga systems use methods such as meditation, devotional practices, contemplation, and ethical living.

Yoga exercises can be helpful to you whether you work out or just walk from the student union to the chemistry building; whether you are as limber as a cat or as stiff as a bicycle; whether you are broad or narrow, old or young. In short, Yoga adapts to your body's fitness level, size, and shape. And if you are athletic, Yoga enhances your other fitness endeavors and helps you avoid injuries. It is a common conditioning regimen for a number of professional sports teams, including members of the Denver Broncos football team, Stanford University's basketball team, and the Ottawa (Canada) Senators' hockey team.[2]

With origins in India as early as 5,000 years ago, Yoga has undergone changes and adaptations over time and has spawned hundreds of different "schools." The school of Yoga we will mainly be concerned with in this book is *Hatha Yoga* (pronounced hut-ha) and its modern offshoots, which emphasize the benefits of Yoga-style exercise.

For us to understand how Hatha Yoga works and the variety of practices that have been incorporated into modern Yoga systems, we need to understand other Yoga schools. And we need to learn about Yoga's rich history and philosophy.

In Chapter 1 we ask, "What is yoga?" and explore the history of Yoga. In Chapter 2 we explore the philosophy of Yoga. Then, in Chapter 3, we focus on the theories of Hatha Yoga. Chapters 4 through 7 are about the exercises of Hatha Yoga: breathing, poses and moving exercises, and also relaxation and meditation. Chapter 8 and Appendix B help you continue your study of Yoga.

I sincerely hope that this text, along with your Yoga class, will inspire you to include Yoga as one of

---

[1] "Yoga is stilling the mind," (my paraphrase) is the second sentence in the famous *Yoga Sūtra* of Patanjali. Georg Feuerstein, *The Yoga-Sūtra of Patanjali: A New Translation and Commentary* (Inner Traditions International, Rochester Vt., 1989).

[2] Ira Dreyfuss, "Athletes Say Yoga Stretches Abilities," *Boulder Daily Camera*, March 17, 2003., and Hurn, *Raleigh Examiner*, September 22, 2009.

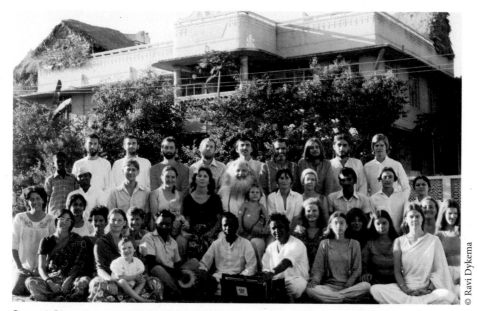

Swami Gitananda (center, with beard) and students in front of Ananda Ashram, Pondicherry, India, 1974. The author (then age 22) is in the back row, far right.

the things you do to stay healthy for the rest of your life!

My Own Story of Finding Yoga

I found Yoga when I was in my early twenties. Before that, in my senior year of high school (1969–70), I took a philosophy class. This class woke me up to the possibility that I wasn't seeing the whole picture—that the world I inhabited, with me as the flawed boy around which the world revolved, was a distortion. I desperately wanted to see more clearly.

In particular, I wanted to understand myself. I had a strong hunch that I was quite different from who I had concluded I was. What started out as a hunch grew into a conviction when I discovered writings by people who felt as I did, people who had studied and practiced systems, such as Yoga, that satisfied their yearnings to see themselves more clearly. Some described a dazzlingly clear kind of seeing that made them feel ecstatic happiness. The writers who most influenced me were Teilhard de Chardin, Alan Watts, Ram Dass, Jack Kerouac, Paramahansa Yogananda, and the author of the *Bhagavad Gita*.

After high school I pursued my quest for self-understanding at Antioch College in Yellow Springs, Ohio. At age 20, in 1972, I traveled to Pondicherry, India, to study Yoga with a renowned teacher, Swami Gitananda.[3] I took Gitananda's six-month teacher training course four times. Swami Gitananda taught traditional Raja Yoga, Tantra Yoga, and Hatha Yoga. In 1974, Gitananda bestowed on me the title *Yogiraj*, which means "master of Yoga."

Over the last 35 years I have maintained a private practice in Yoga therapy. For the last 30 years I have also been a journalist and a magazine publisher covering the fields of holistic health and human potential.

I was an adjunct professor of Yoga at Naropa University in Boulder, Colorado, where I taught for sixteen years (1990 to 2005). My Yoga students, especially those at Naropa University, were and are my main inspiration for writing this textbook. You will find quotes from my Naropa students throughout the book.

A Note on Words Used in This Book

I use the term *yogin* (pronounced yo-ghin) to denote both male and female practitioners of Yoga, although in the Sanskrit language the word means "male practitioner" and the word *yogini* means female practitioner. When I write about a person or a yogin, I alternately use the pronouns his and her.

The word *Yoga* appears in scholarly writings both uncapitalized, as in "yoga," and capitalized, as in "Yoga." In the dictionary it is uncapitalized. I choose, as did the great historian of religion, Mircea Eliade, to capitalize

---
[3] Georg Feuerstein, *Encyclopedia of Yoga*, p. 105, Shambhala Publications, Boston Ma., 1997.

it. This is in keeping with the convention of capitalizing names of other great wisdom teachings such as Buddhism and Taoism.

Using the Footnotes

The footnotes throughout this book offer serious students of Yoga valuable ways to learn more about the subject. They explain where certain ideas in the text came from, pointing you to authoritative writings on Yoga. And they sometimes further explain a word or concept mentioned in the text. Feel free to skip right over the footnotes if reading them breaks your flow or hinders your understanding of the text.

Changes to the Second Edition

I have made numerous changes to the text since I first wrote it in 2005, making it more useful to you. These include a new summary in Chapter 3, numerous updates in the text and in footnotes, new descriptions of Yoga lineages in Chapter 8 to reflect changes to them since 2005, and a completely new Yoga Resources section (Appendix B). You will also find this new color edition easier and more fun to read and use!

Acknowledgments

Writing a book such as this requires many people's efforts in addition to the author's. Therefore I am indebted to a community of others, with whom I will feel forever linked through these pages.

My highest appreciation to my late Yoga Guru Swami Gitananda Giri, who took me on as a disciple when I was 20 and gave me my first opportunities to teach Yoga; also to Meenakshi Devi Bhavanani, who carries on the Gitananda Yoga lineage,

for offering me a fabulous teaching post in Colombo, Sri Lanka, when I was but a pup, and for her ongoing support.

I have been a devoted student of the writings of Georg Feuerstein, Ph.D., for many years and found his work invaluable in the creation of this book. I appreciate Dr. Feuerstein for his kind permission to quote him frequently throughout this volume. This book would never have been written without the seed encouragement of my colleague, Donna Farhi.

I feel great appreciation for my colleagues at other universities who reviewed my manuscript and offered much help, including: Lori J. Head, Idaho State University; Susan Gillis Kruma, University of Pittsburgh; Kate Olafson, Saddleback College, Mission Viejo, CA; Jim Salber, California State University, Chico; and Diane Stevens, Washtenaw Community College, Ann Arbor, Michigan.

My special thanks to Leslie and Dan Goodman for their beautiful photos of the āsanas; also to Crystal Hinton and Tyrone Beverly for their time and awesome talent modeling the poses. And thanks to Mike Speer for his photographic magic with bronze statues, and to Elizabeth Bailey for modeling for the photo on page 140.

For her wonderful illustration and artwork, heartfelt thanks to Kelly Burton. Thanks to Stacey Dykema and Shay Longtain for help with the appendixes, and to Judy Moss for help with the bibliography.

My family lived through deadline after deadline for the three years of this project, and I so appreciate and love them all. Thank you Stacey, Cleo, Kryn and Stephanie.

Finally, thanks to the team of people who produced this book at Cengage and also at Matrix Productions and PreMedia Global, especially my Edition I editor Nedah Rose, and production coordinators Aaron Downey at Matrix (Edition I) and Sushila Rajagopal at PreMedia (Edition II).

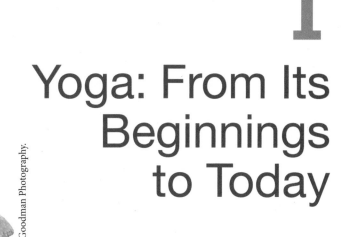
Goodman Photography.

1

Yoga: From Its Beginnings to Today

What Is Yoga?

The word *Yoga* has come to mean many things (Figure 1.1). People who hear the word Yoga may think it refers to an exercise system that originated in India and that is characterized by pretzel-like positions and stretching. Others think Yoga also includes breathing and relaxation practices. Someone who has taken a class in one of the relatively new systems at an athletic club may think Yoga is a sweaty, effortful endeavor designed to build stamina and strength. A person who has been to see a Yoga therapist, perhaps at a health spa, may think Yoga is a complementary healing system[1] for eliminating back pain or helping with recovery from an illness. Still others think Yoga is a religious practice that involves gurus (spiritual authorities) and hymns sung in a foreign language. All of these definitions of Yoga are accurate, and there are many more.

The Sanskrit word *Yoga* derives from the root, "yuj," to yoke, harness, or join together. So Yoga is commonly translated to mean "union."[2] In many

---

[1] Also called complementary and alternative medicine (CAM), and holistic medicine. Sometimes the word *healing* replaces the word *medicine*.

[2] Some other definitions of Yoga are spiritual endeavor—especially the control of the mind and

योग
yo ga

Kelly Burton/Cengage Learning

FIGURE 1.1   "Yoga" written in Sanskrit script.

Yoga traditions, the union referred to is that of your individual self with your universal self. Or, put another way, it means the union of the ordinary you, the you who says, "I think," or "I am reading these words," with the you who is much bigger, much more a part of everything else. This bigger self is sometimes called your "spiritual self," your "true self," or your "soul." The Sanskrit words that connote this union are *jīva-ātman* (living self, individuated self), which unites with *parama-ātman* (supreme self).

A more general description of what is joined or united through Yoga

---

senses, a Hindu tradition of spiritual discipline, self-realization, union with God, and even "separation." Feuerstein, *The Yoga Tradition*.

Meditation Defined

Meditation is the practice of sitting quietly with one's eyes closed or open and focusing attention on one thing, such as the breath, a sound, or an imagined image (for example, the image of the sun). According to many Yoga teachings, as a result of doing a practice like this repetitively one can open and expand one's view and perception.

This expanded perception feels good, reduces stress, and brings one insight into issues such as who one is and what the world is. In all Yoga systems, meditation is a step to *Samādhi* (pronounced sum-ahd-hi), which happens when one's perception is perfectly clear, when one sees oneself and reality completely accurately.

practice is taken from *The Essentials of Yoga* by Sarley and Sarley: "Yoga is . . . designed to balance and unite the mind, body and spirit."[3] A renowned Yoga teacher from India, B.K.S. Iyengar (1918-present) writes in *Yoga, The Path to Holistic Health,* "The primary aim of Yoga is to restore the mind to simplicity and peace, and free it from confusion and distress."[4] Another great Yoga teacher, Swami Vishnudevananda, writes in the foreword to *The Shivananda Companion to Yoga,* "Yoga, the oldest science of life, can teach you to bring stress under control—not only on a physical level, but on mental and spiritual levels too."[5]

You see, defining the word Yoga isn't simple. Most people in the Western world who use the word mean an exercise system. Yet many others refer to a *meditation* system (see Box 1.1) or a spiritual lifestyle.

There really is no handy answer to the question, "What is Yoga?" because Yoga has been evolving and changing throughout its history, and especially recently. Since about 1999, Yoga has rapidly become a more and more popular offering at fitness clubs and recreation centers, colleges, and universities. A 1994 Roper poll, commissioned by *Yoga Journal,*[6] found that 6 million Americans practiced Yoga regularly.

Fourteen years later in 2008 a Harris Interactive Service Bureau survey found that 6.9 percent of U.S. adults, or 15.8 million people, practice yoga, over two-and-a-half times as many as the number stated in the Roper poll.[7]

With so many newcomers to Yoga, the system itself is changing, further complicating the answer to, "What is Yoga?" Teachers adapt their teachings to the people who are showing up for class, and Yoga practitioners who are looking for training as teachers seek schools that present the kind of Yoga they are used to.

This change means that Yoga is morphing into something so different from the traditions from which it arose that Yoga experts who studied the discipline just 30 years ago don't recognize it as Yoga. Veteran journalist Anne Cushman writes in a 2002 *Yoga Journal* article, "Certainly, the form in which Yoga is practiced has altered so radically in the West that it is almost unrecognizable to a traditional Hindu, Buddhist, or Jain practitioner."[8]

[3] Sarley and Sarley, *The Essentials of Yoga,* 4.

[4] Iyengar, Yoga, *The Path to Holistic Health,* 9.

[5] Lidell, *TheSivananda Companion to Yoga,* 7.

[6] Cushman, Anne "The New Yoga," *Yoga Journal,* no. 151, Jan-Feb, 2000.

[7] Harris Interactive Service Bureau Survey, for *Yoga Journal,* Feb 26, 2008.

[8] Cushman, "The New Yoga," *Yoga Journal.*

Some Yoga experts and scholars say that modern fitness-style Yoga is an unfortunate distortion of a valuable tradition. Renowned Yoga scholar Georg Feuerstein writes in an article in *Yoga International* magazine, "If we want to ensure a healthy future for Yoga . . . we must not only look ahead, we must also look back into the past. We must remember Yoga's traditional roots, for without a proper alignment with India's profound spiritual heritage our contemporary Yoga practice is bound to be watered down more and more until it is ineffective as a tool for personal transformation."[9]

Another well-known Yoga teacher, Donna Farhi, writes in the introduction to *Yoga Mind, Body and Spirit*, "Like the botanist who finally breeds the perfect rose only to discover that in the process he has lost the fragrance of the bloom, when we strip Yoga to its mechanics, we also lose something essential. The task of today's teachers and students is to reclaim the essential spirit and intentions behind these practices."[10]

But other leaders in the Yoga community disagree. They say that Yoga has adapted to the needs of people today (by focusing almost exclusively on the body), just as it has adapted for millennia, and they believe that this most recent adaptation is appropriate. Yet a third group of influential teachers says that the popular physical practices are an important entry point into Yoga's broader methods of self-improvement, and that in time many students will become interested in the spiritual and mental aspects of Yoga.[11]

You may wonder what this disagreement among Yoga teachers has to do with your study of Yoga; what does it have to do with your forward bending flexibility, for example? I and many others believe that you, the student, can understand Yoga better and use forward bending poses more effectively if you know why such poses were developed to begin with and how other Yoga practitioners may be using them. When we understand something of Yoga's context, how it has developed over thousands of years into the remarkable systems we have today, we can benefit more from our practice.

The Big Question, "Who Am I?"

The word *Yoga*, you learned earlier, means an exercise system and a method to achieve the union of your individual self with the you who is much bigger, such as your spiritual self, your true self, or your soul, called *parama-ātman*. The methods Yoga has prescribed for achieving that union have varied greatly over the 5,000 years of its history, but the goal, the state of consciousness (which is also called "Yoga,") appears to have been quite consistent: to answer the question "Who am I?" There is even a school of Yoga, *Jnana Yoga* (described later in this chapter), that teaches as its primary practice the continuous asking of this question.

Who am I? Am I my body and its tasting, touching, and smelling? Am I my mind and its thoughts and memories? Am I my dreams and aspirations? Am I what other people think and feel about me? Am I a spiritual being? These are the sorts of questions yogins have been asking for millennia. But to be fair, so have millions of non-yogins. I asked, "Who am I?" when I was a teenager. So did most of my friends. Perhaps you wonder sometimes about who you are, too.

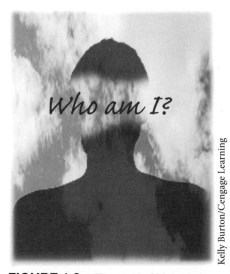

FIGURE 1.2   The goal of Yoga is to answer the question, "Who am I?"

Kelly Burton/Cengage Learning

[9] Feuerstein, "The Lost Teachings," *Yoga International*.

[10] Farhi, *Yoga Mind, Body and Spirit*, xv.

[11] Cushman, The New Yoga, Russell Wild; "Yoga Inc.," both from *Yoga Journal*.

One way people have historically found answers to that question, and satisfied their curiosity, is by looking outside of themselves. They have found answers from religious authority such as that represented by a scripture, a priest, or a dogma. Another way people satisfy their curiosity about who they really are is from parental teaching and example; again, outside of themselves. Yet another way is by adopting the answers common to their society's traditions—still another external source of answers.

But there have been some, in nearly every society, who, seek answers to the question, "Who am I?" from within their own experience.[12] They are saying to their priests and parents and schoolteachers, "What you say makes some sense, but I want to see for myself; I want to *know* with more certainty who I am." These people are called mystics.[13] They all share a doubt that what they have heard or seen is the whole story. That doubt inflames their curiosity and inspires them to explore, to search, to reach into the unknown. In the case of yogins, millions have undertaken this inner exploration. An ancient and modern practice that most captures the spirit of this kind of inner searching is meditation (see Box 1.1). Meditation is the most common practice among most of the old Yoga schools.

You might wonder what these yogins and mystics are exploring—what I mean by "their own experience" or "inner exploration." Please try this exercise before you read on, and I think you will understand better what I mean. Read the whole exercise first, and then try it.

Sit with your feet flat on the floor and your back pretty straight. Close your eyes, and focus on your body. Relax your arms and legs. Relax your lower jaw and your tongue. Now take five slow, deep, easy breaths through your nose, unless it is clogged, in which case breathe through your mouth and nose. For all five breaths sense your body, your sensations of breathing. Afterward, keep sensing your body and open your eyes. Does the world seem any different? Is your vision or hearing any different? Does your body feel different than it did before the exercise? Just notice. Whatever you are experiencing is OK. There is no right way to do this exercise (Figure 1.3).

You may have noticed, as I did when I just did the exercise, that the world does seem a little different afterward. I find it hard to say exactly how it is different. Sharper, maybe, or brighter. Yogins have written that when our world seems to change in these ways, it is really our perception that has changed, not the world. Just imagine what would happen if your perception changed a lot! You might open your eyes after focusing on your breathing and burst into tears at the utter beauty surrounding you. You might see a color as if for the first time, maybe the brilliant green color of the bush outside your window. Here's how a modern mystic and scholar, Ken Wilber, describes one such state:

> Resting in that empty, free, easy effortless witnessing, notice that the clouds are arising in the vast space of your awareness. The clouds are arising within you—so much so, you can taste the clouds, you are one with the clouds, it is as if they are on the inside of your skin, they are so close. The sky and your awareness have become one, and all

---

[12] Alain Daniélou writes in *Yoga, Mastering the Secrets of Matter and the Universe*, "Shaivite philosophy [another name for a school of Yoga] reveals a profoundness of mind which refused to dogmatize or systematize conclusions further than observation would allow them to be verified. Every effort was aimed at developing the human mind's means of perception, of which Yoga techniques became the basis." (p. 10).

[13] Crim, ed., *The Perennial Dictionary of World Religions*, 508.

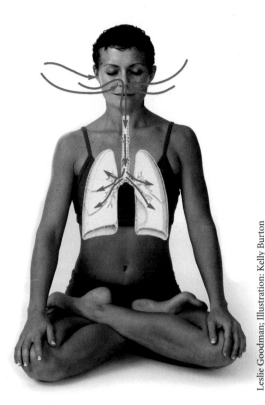

Leslie Goodman; Illustration: Kelly Burton

FIGURE 1.3 Focus on your sensations of breathing.

things in the sky are floating effortlessly through your own awareness. You can kiss the sun, swallow the mountain, they are that close.[14]

An experience such as that described by Wilber answers the question, "Who am I?" When "the sky and your awareness have become one," to reiterate Wilber's image, you are experiencing Yoga.

In ancient India, many people were asking, "Who am I?," and some were finding answers like the one Wilber describes. We know this from Sanskrit writings from that time, such as the *Upanishads* (pronounced oo-pun-ish-uds), which are among the earliest writings on Yoga. The historical record suggests that these "seers," these yogins, developed systems or methodologies to help other people perceive reality directly and fully. Since there were lots of seers, yogins, and inner

explorers using Yoga's methods, these different people with their different needs developed many diverse Yoga systems. No one kind of Yoga worked for everybody, according to some old Sanskrit writings.[15] But whatever Yoga system a person used, the goal was the same: the direct apprehension of the Self, with a capital S. Or, as I like to state this goal in my classes at Naropa University, Yoga helps us see who we are and what the deal is. Put another way, Yoga helps us *really* answer the question, "What's up?"

We're seeing that Yoga was a method to help a person clarify and expand their awareness and their consciousness.

How did Yoga go about changing a practitioner's awareness? It did so in many ways, but one school of Yoga, and the one we are most concerned with in this book, Hatha Yoga, used the body and the breath, along with, of course, the mind, to change awareness. Hatha Yoga's focus on the body was controversial because most previous Yoga schools viewed the body, with its appetites and sensations, as a huge impediment to awakening awareness, an impediment to achieving the goal of Yoga. But Hatha Yoga's founders discovered that a strong and balanced *flow of energy* in one's body, as they put it, improved awareness, and made it clearer and brighter. And a balanced energy flow helped one to control one's mind, enabling one to focus attention on one thing for a long time, which they viewed as a necessary skill for opening one's perception.

Let's fast-forward again to Yoga in the United States today. How did a method to change awareness become a method to strengthen abdominal muscles and reduce stress? The exercises that yogins developed to balance energy in their bodies turn out to impart many other benefits, such as increased stamina, more peaceful

---

[14] Wilber, Foreword, *Talks with Ramana Maharshi*, x.

[15] Feuerstein, *The Yoga Tradition*, 19.

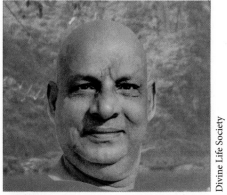

Divine Life Society

PHOTO 1.1 Swami Shivananda of Rishikesh (1887—1963), founder of an influential Hatha Yoga lineage.

BOX **1.2**

Systems, Traditions, or Schools: What Do We Call the Varieties of Yoga?

The diverse teachings of Yoga are called many names. Some words that I (and other writers) use are *system, school,* and *tradition,* all of which mean a coherent body of knowledge that is distinguished from others in significant ways. Another word I use to delineate one type of Yoga from another is *lineage.* This word means "direct descent from an ancestor,"[16] and alludes to the traditional way Yoga knowledge has been passed from generation to generation. This passing of knowledge is called *paramparā* (pronounced, pa-rum-pa-rah'), literally "from one to another." It is a system of oral transmission in which a master of Yoga, a *guru* (pronounced goo-roo) adopts a disciple, a *shishya* (pronounced shish-ya). The master teaches the disciple his or her unique understanding of the Yoga way to awakening. Eventually the disciple may become a master (guru) to new disciples, and on and on.

Yoga lineages are sometimes named after a prominent master, living or dead. An example is Shivananda Yoga, named after Swami Shivananda of Rishikesh, India (1887–1963). Another is Iyengar Yoga, named after B.K.S. Iyengar of Poona, India (1918–present).

Occasionally a person becomes a master, or guru, without having a human teacher, through a process of spontaneous awakening to the truth. They then start a new lineage, or they may claim an affiliation with an old one. An example is Ramana Maharshi of Tiruvannamalai, India (1879–1950), a great adept of *Jnana Yoga*[17] (see below).

sleep, and stronger muscles. So those latter benefits are the ones most Yoga students today are after. And yet, I have heard even the most physically oriented of students say that they feel more contentment since starting their Yoga practice, and they aren't quite sure why. Could it be Yoga's wise ancestors?

Yoga's Beginnings

Yoga developed over thousands of years in response to a perennial hunger in humans to know and understand themselves.

This has led people to create religions, myths, the science of psychology, and mystical systems. Mystical systems are sophisticated methods of investigating one's mind or inner reality. One group of systems of mysticism is called Yoga.

Yoga systems vary greatly from one another. Most people in Western countries are familiar with the posture practice *(āsana)* aspect of Hatha Yoga (for a detailed description of Hatha Yoga, see "Hatha Yoga" later in this chapter). But even that tradition evolved over perhaps 1,000 years from earlier Yoga traditions, and in the company of other evolving Yoga traditions. Like tree branches starting at the trunk and growing toward the sunlight, some long and some short, Yoga schools may be young or old, traditional or modern. All trace their

---

[16] *Webster's New World Dictionary,* Third College Edition.

[17] Maharshi, *Talks with Ramana Maharshi,* xv-xix.

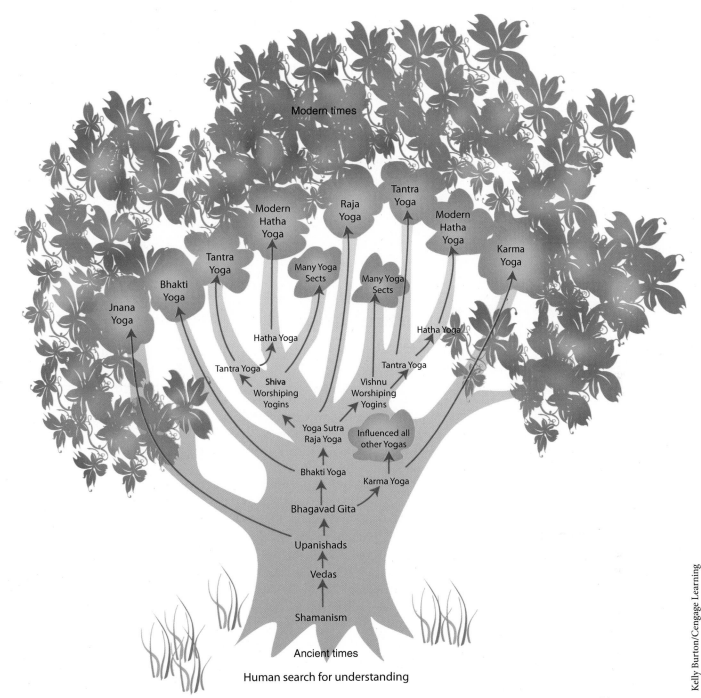

FIGURE 1.4   Like tree branches, some of which are long and some short, Yoga schools may be young or old, traditional or modern.

roots back through the trunk to the human search for understanding. They all are part of the same Yoga tree, and so influence each other (Figure 1.4).

To understand Hatha Yoga and its history, the part of yoga with which we are most concerned in this book, we need to understand at least a little about the other main Yoga systems. I have simplified the list to seven of the most important ones. They are, in approximate order of their historical development, Bhakti Yoga, Mantra Yoga, Karma Yoga, Jnana Yoga, Rāja Yoga, Tantra Yoga, and Hatha Yoga. After you know about these seven Yoga schools, you can better understand the story of Yoga's development from ancient times to the present.

A Bhakti Yoga Exercise

Here is a Bhakti Yoga exercise to try. Sit with your eyes closed and picture the wisest person you can imagine, the most loving and compassionate person you can think of. He or she could be someone you know or someone you hope you might meet someday, a great spiritual figure or a vision of a historical figure such as Jesus. Keep picturing this person as if he or she were sitting in front of you. Hold this image in your mind and send love and appreciation to this person. Continue the exercise for five to ten minutes.

Benefits: An open heart, more compassion for others, and contentment.

Seven of the Most Important Yoga Systems

Bhakti Yoga

The goal of Bhakti (pronounced bhuk-tee) Yoga is communion with or total merging with the divine. The essence of Bhakti Yoga is the act of feeling love and devotion for a divine object or person. Bhakti Yoga is the Yoga most practiced by people in India, and it is at least 3,500 years old. The object of one's love and devotion may be God, a deity such as Krishna (a mythological God-man), Devi (Goddesses), or Vishnu or Shiva (both Hindu Gods). The object of love and devotion could also be a spiritual person, such as a guru, who is a traditional spiritual guide and teacher. Or the object of devotion may be the supreme being, beyond words and concepts.

Bhakti yogins experience the anguish of longing for the divine. It is the Yoga of the heart. Bhakti Yoga practices include singing songs of praise (called *kīrtan* and *bhajana),* meditation on the form of the divine, and acts of service. Bhakti Yoga is closer to Christianity, Judaism, and Islam in temperament than are any of the other Yoga schools.

Please try the exercise in Box 1.3.

Mantra Yoga

Mantra Yoga (pronounced mun-tra) is the Yoga of potent sound. It is the oldest Yoga system, along with Bhakti Yoga, dating back to the oldest scripture in Hinduism, the *Rig Veda,* which was composed about 5,000 years ago. (This date is debated by scholars.)

A mantra is a spiritually charged and powerfully mind-altering sound. The four Vedas and other revered writings of Hinduism were (and still are) traditionally sung or chanted. The words that make up these scriptures are themselves called "mantra," and the phrases from the scriptures are still widely used by mantra yogins.

A mantra could be a single sound, such as "om," which is the most important and widely used power sound in all of Yoga, and connotes the One, or the absolute. A mantra could also be a sentence like "Om namah shivaya," which loosely means, "I merge with the essence of goodness."

Mantras are chanted either out loud or silently in one's mind, sometimes repeated continuously all day, or for hours. Mantras are also used in rituals in temples,, at home altars, and at reflective moments during the day, the way some Christians say grace before eating. In the use of

A Simple Mantra Yoga Meditation

Please try this simple mantra meditation to get a small taste of Mantra Yoga: Sit with your back straight, either cross-legged or in a chair, not leaning back. Close your eyes and relax into your seat, noticing your sensations as you settle earthward. After a minute or two of sensing and relaxing, start repeating over and over to yourself silently, "om, om, om, om. . . ." As you continue this, you may feel as though you are hearing the sound, as opposed to saying it. Let this happen, if it does. When you notice that the sound has stopped, start it again, om, om, om, continuing to repeat om without break, as best you can. Thoughts can come and go. Sounds, memories, scents, body sensations, all can come and go. Just keep hearing or saying om. After five to ten minutes, end the saying of om, relax, and notice your sensations again. After a minute or two, open your eyes.

Benefits: A quieter mind and alertness.

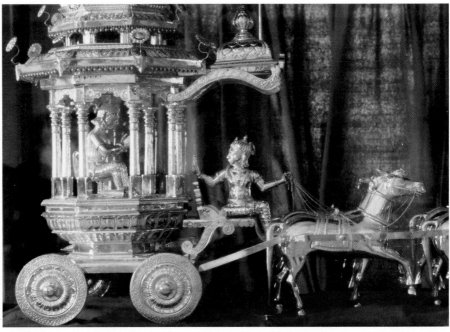

Ravi Dykema

PHOTO 1.2   Lord Krishna (right) instructs Prince Arjuna (left) in the chariot on the battlefield, according to the Yoga scripture, the *Bhagavad-Gītā.*

mantras, Yoga overlaps with *Hinduism,* one of the world's great religions, which is practiced by a majority of Indians. The difference between a practicing Hindu's use of mantra and a mantra yogin's use of mantra is the intensity and purpose of the practice. Whereas a Hindu may use a mantra as a tool for devotion or to influence future events, sort of like a prayer or a magical incantation, a yogin uses mantra to expand and refine his or her awareness, so as to perceive reality more clearly.

Mantra practice constitutes its own Yoga system, but is also included in most of the other schools of Yoga, especially Bhakti Yoga and Tantra Yoga.

Please try the meditation in Box 1.4.

> **BOX 1.5**
>
> # A Simple Karma Yoga Exercise
>
> Here is a simple Karma Yoga exercise to try: Do a favor for someone who will never know who did it, such as put a quarter in someone's expired parking meter, clean someone's dishes, turn in a lost item to the authorities nearest to where it was left, or aright all of the bikes that have fallen over in a bike rack. Notice how you feel as you do this favor, and notice your thoughts as well.
>
> Benefits: Good feelings about yourself, fewer anxious thoughts, and more compassion for others.

Karma Yoga

Karma Yoga (pronounced kar-mah) is the Yoga of selfless action and love, or service to others without desire for reward. Karma Yoga was first taught in the much revered Hindu scripture, the most popular of all ancient Yoga works, the *Bhagavad-Gītā* (200–300 BCE), in which the Lord Krishna instructs the warrior Arjuna on the nature of reality at the beginning of a great battle. He says, "Just as the unwise act attached to action, O Arjuna, the wise should act unattached, desiring the world's welfare."[18]

The goal of the Karma yogin is to perceive reality accurately. The Karma yogin discovers, by acting without desire for results, that she is not the "actor" that she thought she was. Georg Feuerstein, in *The Yoga Tradition*, describes this discovery beautifully: "Karma Yoga is about freedom in action, or the transcendence of egoic motivations. When the illusion of the ego as acting subject is transcended, then actions are recognized to occur spontaneously. Without the interference of the ego, their spontaneity appears as a smooth flow" (p. 48).

Please try the exercise in Box 1.5.

Jnana Yoga

Jnana Yoga (pronounced nyah-nah) is the Yoga of discrimination between the real and the unreal. Jnana Yoga is often called the Yoga of wisdom because "Jnana" means "wisdom."

Jnana Yoga is the teaching contained in the early *Upanishads.* These revered Hindu scriptures were composed between 1500 BCE and 500 BCE. The early Upanishads teach that most of us think that we are individuals with our own independent thoughts, perceptions, and actions, whereas we are actually one with everything; we are one with the ground of reality. An analogy of this oneness used in a later work, *Yoga-Vashishtha* (900 CE),[19] is this: just as the wave is made of ocean water and is one with the ocean, appearing briefly as a separate thing, so are we each one with everything. We mistakenly think of ourselves as individual actors because we see it that way: our senses and minds confirm for us that we are separate people. The Upanishads teach that it is possible for us to see ourselves and reality clearly, as the one reality. To see this reality we need to learn to see beyond our ordinary senses and our ordinary conclusions about who we are.

---

[18] Feuerstein, *The Yoga Tradition*, 63, quote from the *Bhagavad-Gītā*, (3.25).

---

[19] Ibid, 310.

A Jnana Yoga Meditation Practice

Here is a Jnana Yoga meditation practice to try: sit with your back straight, on the floor or in a chair, not leaning back. Sense your legs and your seat and relax into the chair or the floor. Say to yourself, "Who am I, what am I?" Notice what comes next, what sensation, perception, sound, or thought. When you notice some impression, for example, stiffness in your knees, say to yourself, "Not my body"; if you hear voices outside the room, say to yourself, "Not the hearer of sounds"; or, if you notice you have a thought, say to yourself, "Not the thinker." Then re-ask, "Who am I, what am I?" Again notice whatever comes next. When some experience appears, answer the question for yourself with another negation, such as, "Not this itch or the body that itches," or "Not images of me at last weekend's party; not the mind that imagines them." Then re-ask, "Who am I, what am I?" And so on. Continue this exercise for about ten minutes. End the practice by sensing your body again while you relax into the floor. Take a few deep breaths. When you feel ready to encounter the world again, open your eyes.

Benefits: Feelings of lightness, brighter perceptions, calmness, happiness.

The ways to this new seeing taught in the Upanishads are many, but several are dominant: renunciation of the objects we desire, the objects of our senses (this is also called renouncing the world); preparation of one's body and mind through various practices; and meditative practice. The Upanishadic teaching is also called *Vedanta.*

One meditative practice that is used in some Jnana Yoga traditions is self-inquiry, asking, "Who am I?" The most famous modern Jnana yogin was Bhagavan Sri Ramana Maharshi (1879–1950) of South India. Matthew Greenblatt describes Ramana's teachings in the introduction to *Talks with Ramana Maharshi, on Realizing Abiding Peace and Happiness,*[20] "Ramana taught that we exist as the Supreme Self at all times. We need only awaken to this reality by seeking the source of the ego, or 'I-thought,' and abide in the Self that we always are."

Another even more common meditative practice of traditional Jnana Yoga is repeating aloud, or silently to oneself, the sacred syllable, "OM," or "A-U-M." The sound is said to guide the meditator's consciousness to its source, the Absolute, or Brahman. This practice is also used in Mantra Yoga.

Modern Jnana Yoga lineages sometimes dispense with the trappings of tradition and avoid giving a name to what they teach. Their teachings, in contrast to other Yoga systems, may be extremely simple, such as was Ramana Maharshi's method of self-inquiry, asking over and over, "Who am I?"

Please try the meditation in Box 1.6.

Rāja Yoga

Rāja Yoga (pronounced rah-jah), sometimes called Royal Yoga, is known as the Yoga of spiritual kings. This title refers to the Yoga system outlined in the *Yoga Sūtra* by Patanjali, written in about 100 CE.

---

[20] Greenblatt, Introduction, *Talks with Ramana Maharshi,* xvii.

> ### BOX 1.7
>
> # A Basic Rāja Yoga Meditation
>
> Here is a basic Rāja Yoga meditation. Sit cross-legged on the carpet or on a chair with your back straight and your eyes closed. Relax and calm your breathing, letting it become a little deeper and slower. After a few minutes of sensing your breathing, feeling it coming in and going out, pay even closer attention to your exhalation. Breathe out a little more completely, but without any strain, and using very little effort. Your breathing should still feel quite natural and easy. After about five to ten minutes, see if your thoughts have slowed down, and notice if there are any gaps between one thought and another. Come out of this focused state slowly.
>
> Benefits: Greater ease in concentrating, calmness, and joy.

The name "Rāja Yoga" came into use in sixteenth-century India to distinguish Patanjali's system from that of Hatha Yoga, implying the superiority of RājaYoga.[21] Renowned Indologist Alain Danielou has this to say about Rāja Yoga: "This is the highest form of Yoga, all other forms being preparatory."[22]

Yoga experts summarize the purpose of Rāja Yoga fairly consistently: to "become the ruler over (one's) mind" (James Hewitt),[23] "A science of mental discipline" (Satyananda Saraswati),[24] "A path by which the mind and its actions are brought under control (B.K.S. Iyengar).[25]

Another name for this Yoga is the one given to it by Patanjali in his *Yoga Sūtra*: "Ashtanga Yoga." Ashtanga (pronounced ahsh-tan-ga) means "eight limbs," so it is called "eight-limbed Yoga." (See p. 18, "The Yoga of Patanjali," for more on this.) The eighth limb and the goal of Ashtanga/Rāja Yoga is complete identification with the Self, or pure being, which is also called ecstasy *(samādhi)*. The way

Rāja Yoga prescribes to achieve this ecstasy is the seven other limbs, but the primary ones are ethical living, concentration, and meditation.

Rāja/Ashtanga Yoga has evolved into many different schools, including some Hatha Yoga schools, and it has been so influential that some writers claim (I believe erroneously) that it is the one root of all modern Yoga, the oldest and the original Yoga.

The most universal Rāja Yoga exercise, used in every lineage of this tradition, is meditation.

Please try the meditation in Box 1.7.

Tantra Yoga

Tantra (pronounced tahn-trah) Yoga is the Yoga of energy control. The Sanskrit word *tantra* means to extend or stretch out, and refers to the idea that knowledge and understanding are extended by its study. Tantra Yoga developed over hundreds of years in the first half of the first millennium CE. Its goal is the realization of the one Self that is the essence of all beings and all things. Tantra Yoga (also called simply "Tantra") offered a revolutionary new way for the yogin to quest for truth and understanding because Tantra suggested that our bodies, desires, and impulses were expressions of the divine, and therefore useful in our pursuit of divine awareness. This

---

[21] Feuerstein, *The Yoga Tradition*, 37.

[22] Daniélou, Yoga, *Mastering the Secrets of Matter and the Universe*, 90.

[23] Paraphrased from James Hewitt, *The Complete Yoga Book*, 9.

[24] Saraswati, *Yoga from Shore to Shore*, 95.

[25] Iyengar, *Yoga, the Path to Holistic Health*, 14.

contrasted with the attitude of Rāja Yoga, traditional Jnana Yoga, and classical Hinduism, which held that our desires and our bodies were obstacles to our Self-understanding, to our seeing reality clearly. Feuerstein writes, "India's more ascetic—verticalist—traditions have typically looked upon the body as an inconvenience, even an obstacle, to the bliss of freedom. The body and bodily functions fill ascetics of whatever provenance with disgust and horror."[26] In contrast to this renunciate attitude, practitioners of Tantra view their desires, feelings, and worldly involvement, even their sexuality, as aids in their awakening. To them, "the world is the body of the Ultimate Being; women are Shakti (the Goddess) in human guise; sex is the love play between Shiva (God) and Shakti; pleasure is a modification of supreme bliss."[27]

Tantra includes parts of other Yoga systems: devoting oneself to the divine *(bhakti),* chanting power sounds *(mantra),* and visualizing potent symbols *(yantra).* Of all the Yoga systems, Tantra Yoga is the most complex, and certainly the most misunderstood. One common misunderstanding is that Tantra concerns itself primarily with sexuality. Traditional Tantra did include among its many sects some that used sexual intercourse *(maithunā)* in a ritual context. These were called "left-hand-path Tantra" or *Vama Marga* Tantra. But even for yogins in the left-hand sects, the sexual ritual was a small part of their practice.[28]

Incidentally, there is a Buddhist version of Tantra that is related to Tantra Yoga, and which developed at the same time. It is better understood in the West than Tantra Yoga because

of the diaspora of Tibetan Buddhist monks that resulted from the invasion of Tibet by the Chinese in 1950. Buddhist Tantra is also known as *Vajrayana* (diamond vehicle).

Tantra Yoga spawned a school of Yoga called Hatha Yoga, which is now considered a distinct Yoga system, and is described in the next section

Please try the exercise in Box 1.8.

Hatha Yoga

Hatha Yoga is the Yoga of balanced body energy. "Hatha" (pronounced, hut-ha) means "forceful." But I have called it the Yoga of balanced body energy because of another esoteric translation of "Hatha": "Ha" equals sun, and "tha" (pronounced t-ha) equals moon, which metaphorically refers to the right and left flows of energy united in the human body. Hatha Yoga practice stimulates and balances these two energies so that a yogin can clear his or her lens of perception and see reality.

Hatha Yoga developed as an offshoot of Tantra Yoga[29] in the first half of the first millennium CE. The historic innovation of Hatha Yoga, as with Tantra Yoga, was that the yogin's body was seen as a continuum with his or her mind, so that a change in both body and mind was viewed as a way to become free from misconceptions and see clearly. Hatha Yoga sought to so transform the yogin's body that it was called a divine body *(divya-sharira)*[30] that didn't suffer from disease or discomfort. In addition, this divine body was said to have super-sensory powers—seeing, hearing, touching, intuiting—and paranormal abilities *(siddhi),* somewhat like those used by wizards in the Harry Potter books and movies. Partly because of the allure of these

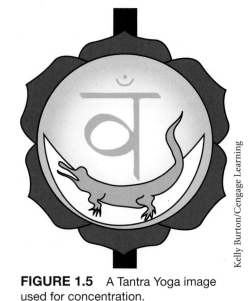

Kelly Burton/Cengage Learning

FIGURE 1.5   A Tantra Yoga image used for concentration.

[26] Feuerstein, *Tantra, the Path of Ecstasy,* 224–225.

[27] Ibid. 227.

[28] Ibid. xiii–xiv.

[29] Saraswati, *Teachings of Swami Satyananda Saraswati,* 211.

[30] Feuerstein, *Tantra,* 39.

BOX 1.8

A Tantra Yoga Breath Exercise

A simple Tantra Yoga breath exercise can illustrate for you the kind of concentration that is common in Tantra Yoga. Sit cross-legged with your back straight, or if that requires strain, sit in a chair without leaning back. Close your eyes and focus on your sensations for a few minutes. Then focus on your breath, feeling your sensations of breathing in your nose, in your chest and back, and in your belly. Start counting as a way to time your in and out breaths, six counts in, six counts out (or four counts in and out). If counting your breath remains uncomfortable for more than three breaths, just breathe in and out more deeply than usual, without counting. After a little while, add a visualization: while breathing in, picture warm energy moving up in your body, while breathing out, picture cool energy moving down in your body. Now add a sound to all that you are doing: on your in-breath, think, "ahh-hhh." On your out-breath, think, "eeeeeee." Continue this practice for five to ten minutes, only if it feels easy and comfortable. It is especially important to keep feeling your sensations of breathing, or come back to those sensations when you discover that your mind has wandered. To end, return to automatic, natural breathing and sense your body for a little while. Then slowly open your eyes.

Benefits: Feeling increased energy and alertness, yet combined with calmness and a feeling of being centered.

powers, and because of the danger to yogins of becoming too body-preoccupied, Hatha Yoga came under attack early in its development as decadent and degenerate. To some extent, this criticism continues to this day.

Hatha Yoga's body-changing methods are considered incomplete as a mystical path in the three most important old Sanskrit works on the subject[32] and in some modern lineages. In these works Hatha Yoga is called a "stairway" to Rāja Yoga, which completes it by providing mental and meditative practices. Yet this perspective is not universal to all Hatha Yoga lineages, because from its beginnings Hatha Yoga has, like Rāja Yoga, included concentration, meditation, and the final goal of ecstatic awareness (samādhi).

The primary Hatha Yoga methods in all the traditional schools are

purification practices, breath control (especially the ability to suspend the breath for a long time), and body movements and positions (āsanas, or poses). These practices impart a kind of super-fitness, as well as producing states of concentration and meditation. These practices were, taken together, designed to arouse an energy that was usually unavailable to people, an energy that could propel one into higher states of awareness. This energy is called *kundalinī shakti*, or coiled energy. I discuss this further in Chapter 3.

Modern Hatha Yoga is often simplified to a limited number of choreographed movements and static positions that create muscle strength and elasticity called *āsanas*. Although āsanas originated in a much larger context, they are so effective that by themselves, as āsana yoga, they provide people with an excellent way to become healthy and fit.

Please try the exercise in Box 1.9.

---

[31] *Gheranda-Samhita, Hatha-Yoga-Pradipika,* and *Shiva-Samhita.*

BOX **1.9**

A Hatha Yoga Exercise

Please try this Hatha Yoga exercise to experience a bit of the "balanced energy" that I have been describing. Assume a dog-like position on a blanket or carpeted floor. With your knees about hip-width apart and your arms shoulder-width, hang your head and relax your weight into the floor. Now curve your back slowly in a sway fashion while lifting your head, keeping your arms straight and your weight centered between your hands and knees. Next, slowly move your back toward the opposite curve, that is, arching your back and dropping your head down between your arms. Your mid-back is rising toward the ceiling as you curve it. Continuously repeat this pattern, swaying, head up; arching, head down [1.3 and 1.4]. After a few of these, add an in-breath as you sway your back, and an out-breath as you arch your back, adjusting your speed so your breathing is easy. Please don't work hard or strain at this. Take it easy. And, this is very important, pay close attention to your sensations—your breathing, your body—the whole time, as best you can. After about ten to fifteen of these movements, stop and remain on your hands and knees for a few more breaths. Then assume a resting position and keep sensing your body. Also notice how you feel as you get up from this practice.

Benefits: Feeling more of whatever state your body was in before you performed the exercise: more tired, more alert, hungrier, and so on. The exercise turns off your mind a little and turns on your body, so you can feel it more directly. You may feel like doing more Yoga exercises because you're more in tune with what your body wants, and you've teased it with a little bit of exercise. Also, feeling more in tune usually gives you more energy.

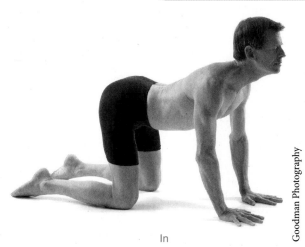
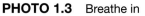
Goodman Photography

PHOTO 1.3   Breathe in

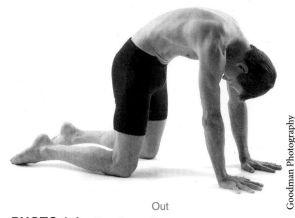
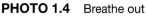
Goodman Photography

PHOTO 1.4   Breathe out

What Is the Same in All Yoga Systems?

All the systems of Yoga agree on two things: One, the goal of Yoga practice is full awareness of one's true Self (samādhi or *Brahman*). Two, an essential means to that goal, an essential practice, is ethical and moral living. Whether we are investigating Jnana Yoga, Mantra Yoga, Rāja Yoga, or Hatha Yoga, all teach these two ideas.[32] About many other matters the

---

[32] Feuerstein, *Yoga Tradition*, 28.

The Shaman

The word shaman comes from a Siberian word and describes a man, or less often a woman, who changes his or her consciousness so that she or he can see, hear, and touch things that ordinary people can't. In other words, the shaman can travel in his or her mind to extraordinary worlds with landscapes, plants, animals, and people, all of which are considered to be in the spirit realm. The shaman travels to the spirit world on behalf of an ill person or for the benefit of a community. (In the case of Native Americans, the terms "medicine man" or "medicine woman" are sometimes used as synonyms for "shaman.") The system that a shaman uses to change his or her consciousness and to affect the spirit world, and thus to affect the ordinary human world, is called "Shamanism." The words *Shaman* and *Shamanism* have come to be used for practices that arose in many parts of the world independently from the Shamanism of Siberia.

systems, or schools, differ. Some say the journey is hard (Hatha Yoga); others say it is easy (some sects of Jnana Yoga). Some schools prescribe meditation and chanting (Bhakti Yoga); others teach hundreds of complicated exercises (Tantra Yoga). A number of systems dismiss our bodily experience as *impediments* to awakening. Others, like Tantra and Hatha Yoga, see our bodies as essential to awakening. Read more about this in Chapter 3.

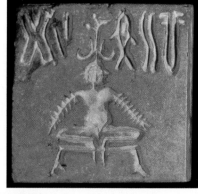

PHOTO 1.5 Steatite seal from Mohenjo-Daro, a city in India before 2800 BCE, which is thought to depict a yogi.

Borromeo / Art Resource, NY

A Short History of Yoga

How Old Is Yoga?

The answer depends on what you mean by Yoga. If you mean Yoga poses (āsanas), then the answer is about 1,000 to 1,500 years old because that is the commonly estimated age of Hatha Yoga, in which developed the system of body postures called āsanas. If you mean the whole of the yoga tradition, then the answer is it is very old indeed, as you'll see.

Yoga's history is integrally linked to that of the dominant religion on the Indian subcontinent: Hinduism. Yoga and Hinduism share many

of the same sacred writings, and Yoga-like practices are used by many Hindus, such as sitting quietly and holding a single thought in one's mind. The difference between Yoga and Hinduism is that Yoga is a mystical system that doesn't require belief in God or a supreme being (except in the case of Bhakti Yoga, the Yoga of devotion). A yogin can even *doubt* that there is such a thing as God and still derive benefit from practicing Yoga. Hinduism, on the other hand, is a religion. It is a diverse religion with many divisions or sects, which makes it hard to generalize about beliefs. Yet most Hindus believe in God or a supreme being, and much of the benefit to them from practicing their religion derives from their beliefs. We will explore this subject of Gods, religion, and Yoga more in Chapter 2.

The Earliest Roots of Yoga

Scholars surmise that Yoga-like practices existed among ancient shamans in what is now India and Pakistan. Scholars have dated Shamanism to around 25,000 BCE, pre-dating written history. Shamanism's similarity to Yoga is in its mind-altering technologies and in the way it was passed on from one person to another, a process called initiation. Shamanism is dissimilar to Yoga in its focus on engaging the spirit world in order to *accomplish something,* such as to heal a person or a community. The yogin, in contrast, focuses on his or her *own transformation* into a fully awake state. Whether this awake state includes spirit beings is unimportant to the yogin. The yogin often withdraws from other people to pursue this goal, in contrast to the shaman's role as a spiritual leader in his or her community. The most fundamental difference between Shamanism and Yoga is that whereas the shaman is looking outward into the world of spirits, the yogin is looking inward. Georg Feuerstein writes in *The Yoga Tradition*:

> The condition of illumination, or enlightenment, is to the yogin what the magical journey into other realms is to the shaman. Both experiences represent a radical departure from conventional reality and consciousness. Both have a profoundly transformative effect. Yet only the yogin, who travels inward, discovers the ultimate futility of all journeying, because he realizes that he is never traveling outside the very reality that is the goal of his spiritual odyssey.[33]

The next era of Yoga's evolution was the time of the four Vedas, the first of which, the *Rig-Veda,* was written before 3,000 BCE. (This date is debated.) The Yoga-like practices in the Vedas are meditation, chanting sacred hymns (mantras), and acts of self-sacrifice for the purpose of surrendering the ego. Among these practices, the one that is the most central to all later Yoga systems is meditation. Feuerstein calls meditation the "fulcrum of Yoga."[34]

Later, while a great river, the Saraswati, was slowly drying up in North India,[35] displacing the centers of Vedic civilization eastward to the Ganges River and its tributaries, the Vedic religious teachings were undergoing a transformation, too. The religious elite, the brahmins, conducted complex rituals on behalf of worshipers. As the rituals became more sophisticated and the priesthood became more exclusive, people longed for a more immediate experience of the Divine. Many of them turned to unorthodox teachers of mystical paths that promised direct contact with the Divine within, with one's true nature. This pattern seems to reoccur a number of times in Yoga's history, as people's impulse to explore themselves breaks out of the constraints imposed by those who try to control people's beliefs and maintain an established order. Among these unorthodox teachers of mystical paths were the writers of the early Upanishads (literally, "To sit down close to one's teacher").

The Vedic culture was preoccupied with the precise execution of ritual sacrifice, especially using a small fire and numerous symbolic objects such as milk, rice, flowers, and fruit. The innovation of the Upanishadic sages was that they described a way to perform an inner sacrifice symbolically, as in this passage from the *Kaushitaki-Brahmana-Upanishad,* "Verily, as long

---

[33] Feuerstein, *Yoga Tradition,* 127.

[34] Ibid., 138.

[35] Feuerstein, Kak, & Frawley, *In Search of the Cradle of Civilization: New Light on Ancient India.*

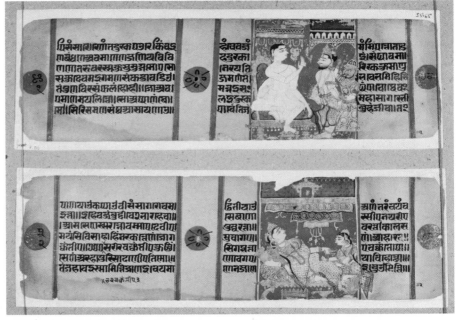

Borromeo / Art Resource, NY

PHOTO 1.6   An ancient manuscript, part of the Kalapsutra. Late 14th century.

as a person is speaking, he is unable to breathe. Then he is sacrificing the breath to speech. Verily, as long as a person is breathing, he is unable to speak. Then he is sacrificing the speech to the breath. . . . Understanding this, the ancestors did not offer the fire sacrifice literally.[36] This sort of inner worship was revolutionary around 1,000 BCE because it offered a way for anyone to realize his or her Self. This true Self, or fundamental Self, the Upanishadic sages wrote, is the same as the reality underlying everything, called Brahman, the absolute. Furthermore, this Self, this absolute, is unquestionably real, is unbounded by time or space, is free, is never born

and never dies, and is intensely blissful. This idea that the Self *is* the absolute became the philosophical basis for most of the Yoga systems that have evolved into modern forms.

Out of these separate but interrelated influences grew the different systems of Yoga that exist today, containing the common practices of meditation, ethical living, and withdrawal from the world of sensual enjoyment.

The Yoga of Patanjali: Classical Yoga and the *Yoga Sūtra*

Patanjali lived around 100 to 200 CE, based on scholars' estimates of the date of his famous work, the *Yoga Sūtra* (literally, Yoga thread). Nothing

---

[36] Feuerstein, *Yoga Tradition*, 125.

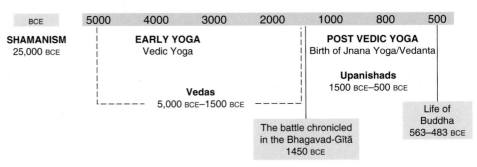

| BCE | 5000 | 4000 | 3000 | 2000 | 1000 | 800 | 500 |

SHAMANISM 25,000 BCE

EARLY YOGA Vedic Yoga

POST VEDIC YOGA Birth of Jnana Yoga/Vedanta

Upanishads 1500 BCE–500 BCE

Vedas 5,000 BCE–1500 BCE

Life of Buddha 563–483 BCE

The battle chronicled in the Bhagavad-Gītā 1450 BCE

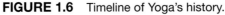

FIGURE 1.6   Timeline of Yoga's history.

BOX **1.11**

The Upanishads

This genre of Hindu literature is considered sacred revelation *(shruti)* that refines, but does not contradict, the earlier Vedic teachings. In fact, the Upanishadic teaching is called *Vedanta,* meaning "the end of the Vedas." Numbering over 200, the Upanishads were written by sages as long ago as 1,500 BCE and as recently as the twentieth century CE. The early Upanishads are considered to be the source of Jnana Yoga.

else about Patanjali is known. Some scholars of Indian tradition have equated him with a grammarian (scholar of grammar) of the same name who lived around four hundred years earlier, but the majority opinion separates the two.

Patanjali's *Yoga Sūtra* became the authoritative work on Yoga and remains the most-quoted Sanskrit writing on the subject in Yoga classes today. The *Yoga Sūtra* is considered a compilation and reformulation of Yoga, and not an original exposition. Thus the Yoga practices that the *Sūtra* describes can be assumed to have existed for many years prior to its writing. In fact, the *Katha Upanishad* (400 BCE), the earliest work in which Yoga became a recognizable tradition in its own right, teaches that Yoga is "the steady holding of the senses. Then one becomes attentive." [37] This is very similar to the opening lines of the *Yoga Sūtra,* which

I will discuss below. Another Upanishad, the *Maitrayaniya Upanishad* (200 BCE), includes a "six-limbed" method that corresponds closely to Patanjali's "eight-limbed" system.

The *Yoga Sūtra* was the most comprehensive and organized Yoga work of its day, and it became hugely influential. Because of it, Yoga became and still is one of the "six viewpoints" *(shat-darshana)* of orthodox Hinduism: Yoga, Samkhya, Mımamsa, Vedanta, Nyaya, and Vaisheshika. All six offer methods for understanding one's True Nature, but Yoga is the most elaborate and the most practical.

Patanjali called his organization of Yoga's practical steps "eight-limbed Yoga" *Ashtangayoga* (pronounced ash-tan-ga yo-ga (see Box 1.12). It later was referred to as Rāja Yoga (royal Yoga). One modern Hatha Yoga teacher, Sri K Pattabhi Jois of Mysore, India, calls his system "Ashtanga Yoga." It is known for its

---

[37] Ibid., 35.

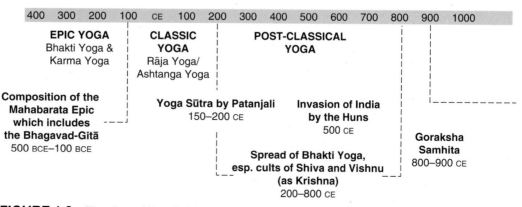

FIGURE 1.6   Timeline of Yoga's history. *(Continued)*

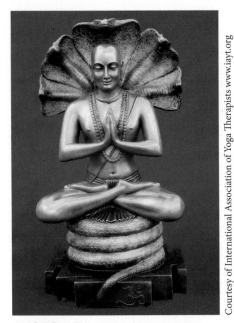

Courtesy of International Association of Yoga Therapists www.iayt.org

PHOTO 1.7   Statue of Patanjali sitting on a coiled cobra.

The Eight Limbs of Rāja Yoga

1. Yama (pronounced yah-ma): the "moral disciplines" of nonharming, truthfulness, nonstealing, chastity, and nongreediness. These relate to one's social relationships.

2. Niyama (pronounced nee-yah-ma): the "self restraints" of purity contentment, austerity, self-study, and devotion to the lord. These relate to one's inner life.

3. Āsana (pronounced ah´-sa-na): firm seat, meaning a seated posture that is motionless and easy. Patanjali did not mean, according to many sources, the many poses that are part of modern Hatha Yoga. (A notable exception is Eliade in *Patanjali and Yoga*.[38])

4. Prānāyāma (pronounced prah-nah-yah-ma): breath control, especially breath suspension.

5. Pratyāhāra (pronounced pra-tya-haa-ra): withdrawal from the objects of one's senses, which includes visions of such objects in one's mind.

6. Dhāranā (pronounced dha´-ra-nah´): concentration, or fixing one's mind on a point in one's body or on a divine form within one's body or outside of it.

7. Dhyāna (pronounced dhy-ah´-na): meditation, which here means the effortless continuation of concentration, of one-pointed focus, such that the object of concentration fills the whole space of one's awareness.

8. Samādhi (pronounced sa-mah´-dhi): ecstasy, or identification with the object of meditation such that the self disappears.

---

athletic intensity and is different from traditional Ashtanga Yoga, which emphasizes meditation.

Patanjali emphasizes the importance of the last three of the eight limbs, namely concentration, meditation, and ecstasy. Patanjali writes, "These three are more direct aids to experience than the five limbs previously

described.[39] Perhaps for this reason Rāja Yoga is often described by scholars or Yoga experts as the Yoga of meditation, or the Yoga of mental control.

Viewed historically, Patanjali's compilation of Yoga is unusual in its teaching that one's living self (*prakriti*) and one's spiritual essence

---

[38] Ibid., 135.

[39] Prabhavenanda, *How to Know God, the Yoga Aphorisms of Patanjali*, 177 (Sūtra 3,7).

| 1100 | 1200 | 1300 | 1400 | 1500 | 1600 | 1700 | 1800 |

MEDIEVAL YOGA

Begining of the Muslim invasion of India
1200 CE

Tantra Yoga and Hatha Yoga
900–1700 CE

British interest in Orientalism. First English translation of Bhagavad Gītā and other scriptures
1785

Hatha Yoga-Pradipika
1300 CE

Yoga Upanishads
1300–1400 CE

Gheranda Samhita
1650 CE

Shiva Samhita
1600–1700 CE

FIGURE 1.6   Timeline of Yoga's history. *(Continued)*

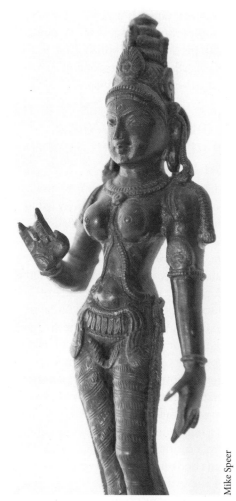

Mike Speer

PHOTO 1.8 In the era of Tantra, the body was no longer considered an obstacle to spiritual experience. Instead, the body was viewed as an asset, as depicted in this bronze statue of the divine as female, inspired by a 13th century style of sculpture.

(*purusha*) are distinct from each other. In other words, Patanjali says that to reach full awareness, the yogin must overcome his or her nature and identify with that which is beyond nature and the world of form. This teaching is called dualism.

In contrast to this, the dominant outlook of the Yoga that preceded Patanjali (pre-classical Yoga) and the Yoga that followed him (post-classical Yoga) was one of nondualism. In the much older Jnana Yoga taught in the early Upanishads, for example, the fully awake yogin discovers that he or she is the Brahman, the supreme Reality, pure consciousness. The yogin discovers that his or her former sense of being separate from other people, from things and from the Supreme, was an illusion. Nondualism such as this is also dominant in the later philosophies of Tantra Yoga and Hatha Yoga.[40]

Patanjali's *Yoga Sūtra* became a central inspiration for nearly all subsequent Yoga systems. But Patanjali's influence was blended with elements from Tantra, and that made a world of difference.

A New Era of Befriending the Body, Tantra Yoga

The powerful human impulse that flowered so spectacularly in India within Yoga and Hindu mysticism was the impulse to know. The perennial

---
[40] Feuerstein, *Yoga Tradition*, 311.

question that the seekers, saints, swamis (holy men), and sages asked was, "Who am I, really?" The answer many of them arrived at through awesome acts of will (austerities), painful sacrifice (renunciation of sense pleasures), and devotion and love was, "I am not my body. I am not my feelings and dreams. I am not my mind or my thoughts. I am not my blissful spiritual experiences. I am consciousness-bliss, I am the stuff of everything, I am the ātman, the self."[41] This spiritual strategy—austerities, renunciation, and devotion—lasted for thousands of years in numerous forms, as you have learned. The yogins and Hindu sages of these times mainly believed that their ordinary human needs, wants, and desires would keep them preoccupied with worldly concerns, identified with their egos, and bound in suffering because they would be cut off from their source of fulfillment, the splendorous Reality they had heard about and yearned to know.

But this strategy and philosophy doesn't entirely make sense. If I am one with my True Self and with the Absolute, and if the Absolute is the ground of everything, then isn't the Absolute in my body, in my attraction to another's body, in my other feelings and thoughts? If everything—me, the universe—whirls around in perfect

---
[41] This is an approximation of a poem by Shankara (788–822 CE), the celebrated teacher of the non-dual Upanishadic wisdom called *Advaita Vedanta*.

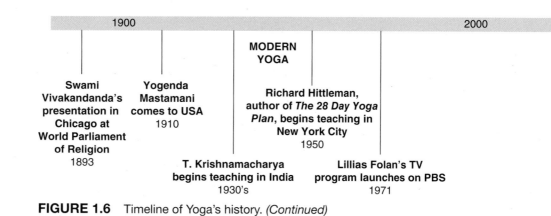

FIGURE 1.6   Timeline of Yoga's history. *(Continued)*

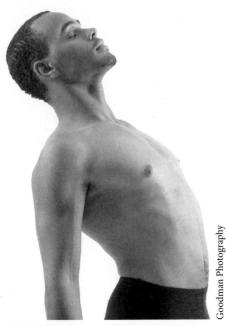

Goodman Photography

PHOTO 1.9 Meditation is still a central part of the practice of Yoga poses (āsanas).

order (it is all the Absolute), as so many ancient sages assert, then isn't my body part of that perfect spin? Do I really have to abandon pleasure to have spiritual bliss?

These are the sorts of questions we might assume the founders of Tantra Yoga asked (the Yoga of energy, also called, simply, Tantra). Their answer? We can *integrate* our spiritual aspirations with our worldly lives. We can integrate our desire for fun with our desire for wisdom. This idea may sound simple, but the methods the Tantra yogins developed were complex and difficult, and they required, as do all Yoga systems, a solid grounding in moral and ethical living for the techniques to be safe and effective.

Tantra Yoga theory teaches that our bodies and our minds are one continuum. Each contributes to the yogin's state of awareness. A healthy body helps one concentrate on a single object for a long time, as in meditation. And a quiet mind helps heal one's body. Modern medical researchers' studies indicating that many illnesses are stress-related are bearing this out. But Tantra yogins discovered, as did yogins before them, that practitioners of Yoga could become super-healthy and extra-vibrant. Such super-vibrancy brightens awareness, makes concentration more effective, and increases the yogin's chances of slipping into meditation (which is when concentration becomes effortless). The central method in Tantra of inducing the energized state of vibrancy is to undergo extensive purification and then to arouse a potent energy that is usually dormant in peoples' bodies called *kundalinī shakti* (coiled energy, or Goddess energy). This energy is then directed via intense concentration and breath control into the center of the yogin's spine. As the energy rises in his or her spine it passes through and opens the seven subtle energy centers called *chakras* (literally, wheels). Once the chakras are open, the yogin is in samādhi, is perceiving with crystal

clear awareness, is in ecstasy. Or put another way, the yogin's self is joined with his or her Self, which is *the* Self of everything and everyone, ātman joined with *parama-ātman*.

Contemporary Yoga: Hatha Yoga and Āsana Yoga

The complexity of Tantra Yoga and its conflict with Hindu orthodoxy led to the development of a simplified version of Tantra's body-transforming methods. Much of Tantra Yoga's theory and practice are retained within Hatha Yoga, especially the importance of purification, the arousal of kundalinī shakti, and the opening of the energy centers, or chakras (for more on Hatha Yoga, see Chapter 3). Some of traditional Tantra's ritualism and elaborate mantras were abandoned by Hatha yogins, while they expanded upon the strengthening and body-conditioning practices that prepared the Tantra yogin's body for the high-voltage flows of energy (shakti). These practices included many poses or positions that the yogin moved through or held, called āsanas. In the last sixty years, many yogins have further simplified Hatha Yoga to a system of from fifty to about two hundred āsanas and around four to eight breath control practices. Yet further simplification (in the last forty years) has resulted in Yoga systems with as few as twenty-six poses and two breathing exercises.[42]

Yoga has evolved and adapted over thousands of years to humanity's passionate desire for self-understanding. It is still adapting. Traditional comprehensive Yoga systems exist today in many places around the globe (see "Resources" in Appendix B). Yoga's renowned flexibility and capacity to reinvent itself has even enabled it to adapt to the needs of modern out-of-shape and stressed-out college students!

---

[42] Choudhury, *Bikram's Beginning Yoga Class*, xi.

Goodman Photography

2

Yoga Philosophy

The Goal of Yoga

Men and women who have experienced the goal of Yoga describe an experience that is "beyond words." Joseph Campbell, renowned historian of religion and myth, said, "The fundamental thought in the Oriental philosophical world is that the mysterious, ultimate truth, that which you seek to know, is absolutely beyond all definition. All categories of thought, all modes of imaging fall short of it."[1]

Yet those who have felt their minds disappear and who have seen clear light pervade everything feel an urge to *tell* others about it. That urge to share a joy that knows no bounds, which the seeker has discovered via a journey into nonordinary consciousness through Yoga, or through singing hymns in church, or through encountering awesome beauty in nature, is the creative fire behind all religions and all mystical systems. Although they may sit alone in rapture for a while, people who have felt the Holy Ghost enter them, or who have felt the grace of God flowing in and around them, or who have lived five minutes of perfect ecstasy will feel a generosity—some have called it love— that they yearn to share with other people.

[1] Campbell, *Myths of Light, Eastern Metaphors of the Eternal,* 6.

So they *do* use words, inadequate though they may be. And those words provide us with a written record that reveals a vibrant and influential system of philosophy. Yoga philosophy is available today not only in books, but also in living teachings that have been passed on through the ages "from mouth to ear" in Yoga lineages.

Describing the goal of Yoga, which is the central idea around which all Yoga philosophy revolves, is like describing to someone who

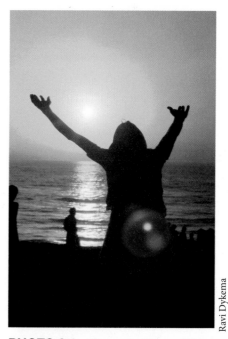

Ravi Dykema

PHOTO 2.1   The experience of Yoga must be felt. It is hard to describe.

23

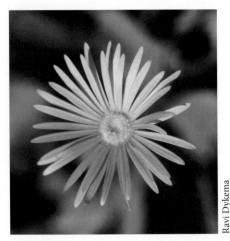

Ravi Dykema

PHOTO 2.2   The flower that was red earlier would appear to you as black and white, even though in reality it was still red.

has never gone swimming how it feels to leap into a shimmering blue swimming pool on a steamy-bright day [2.1]. Or, it is like describing the taste of an orange to someone who has only eaten bread all her life. Or, it is like describing the feelings you had and the rhythms you heard at a rock concert to someone who has only listened to bluegrass music on a clock radio. But I will give it a try.

The Ordinary vs. the Extraordinary vs. the Out of This World

The goal of Yoga is to wake up, to part the veils that obscure your view, and to see yourself and reality as they really are. Ancient yogins have described the reality *they* experienced, but haven't said that *we* must see the same thing. They point the way for others to follow in their footsteps, so to speak, and for those seekers to find out for themselves what lies beyond the orbit of ordinary thoughts and conclusions.

Don't be distressed if you don't know what sort of extraordinary experience I am alluding to. The reason that few people have experienced their big "S" Self, their parama-ātman, is because it is not easy to do.

Consciousness, which is our viewer, our camera through which we perceive ourselves, gets stuck easily. Consciousness gets stuck on a particular channel, like a television channel. In that stuck "channel-land," everything you experience makes sense and serves to confirm your ideas about reality. As an example, let's imagine you live in a black and white world. If you saw a red flower one day as you rode past on your bike, you might stare for a moment with wide eyes, your breath catching in your throat. But quickly your mind would assemble an explanation, such as: it wasn't really red because you were temporarily dreaming. Or it wasn't really red because

your optic nerve must have misfired somehow, and the colored flower was just a trick of brain chemistry. Or it wasn't really red because when you think about the flower moments later as you ride along, you see it in the familiar black and white in your mind's eye. You may even pass the same plant later in the day, and the flower that was red earlier would *appear to you* as black and white, even though in reality it was still red [2.2].

That is how our minds work, according to Yoga philosophy. Here is another explanation using a classic analogy from the Yoga literature: we think we are a wave. We don't see that we are the ocean water appearing for a time as a wave. We base our mistaken belief on the evidence of our senses: we *see* other waves nearby. We *hear* other waves sloshing and whispering. We can *feel* our own wave-like shape and size, which stays consistent day after day. And most important, we have our *own thoughts*. We *think* as a separate wave would think. We say, "*my* froth, *my* speed, *my* steepness, *my* wants, *my* special waviness."

The *Yoga-Vashishtha* says, "What is this idea that 'I exist?' Every single being and thing has arisen from consciousness. Who is the 'I' who is, as it were, a minutest fragment of the Absolute?"[2] It continues a few stanzas later, "He who sees the Self abiding in all beings and all beings in the Self, and he who sees that the Self is not an 'I,' not an ego, he truly sees. Just as the water of waves of different shapes is always the same, so is the Self also in the beings of a desert caravan, or also in the beings of the golden Himalayas [mountains in Tibet]. Just as multitudes of different waves roll in the same ocean, similarly all the beings in the golden Himalayas or in the caravans are really the supreme Self."[3]

---

[2] Feuerstein, *The Yoga Tradition,* 307, stanza 26.
[3] Ibid., p. 310, stanzas 60–62. I have slightly edited Feuerstein's translation from the Sanskrit.

BOX 2.1

Yoga Is Only One of Many Mystical Traditions

Yoga is one of many ways in which humans have understood themselves and the universe. Most major religions include mystical brotherhoods and sisterhoods. Yoga could be seen as a mystical tradition within Hinduism. Other mystical traditions within major religions are Taoism from China; Zen Buddhism from Japan; Christian mysticism (one branch of which is the Essenes), originally from the Middle East; Sufism from all parts of the Islamic world; and Jewish Kabbalah, originally from the Middle East.

The Core Questions

The goal of Yoga is the answer to the question, *"Who am I, really?"* That question and its answer are at the core of Yoga philosophy; all the Yoga systems formed and grew because people have been passionately interested in this question for thousands of years. As people experimented with ways of overcoming their inclination to think of and to see themselves as separate and unique, they discovered a lot about humans. They learned about their minds, their wants, their fears, their hearts, and their bodies. These discoveries make up the other important part of Yoga philosophy—the answer to the question, *"What is the nature of human minds and bodies and how, specifically, can one 'wake up'?"*

Yoga Morals and Ethics

Each system of Yoga came up with a different answer to the question, "Who am I?" We can summarize Yoga's many methods for waking people up into two broad categories: One, Yoga practice *prepares the container.* It changes a person so that they become "riper" and more inclined to have spiritual experiences—the kinds of experiences that answer the question, "Who am I?" Second,

Yoga practice *induces in a person peak experiences:* nonordinary expanded, or supra-sensory states of awareness.

In the first category are teachings about morals and ethics. These teachings are common to all Yoga traditions (see Chapter 1, "What Is the Same in All Yoga Systems?"), so we can presume that ancient yogins considered an ethical and purified lifestyle to be an essential preparation for the kind of training that leads to expanded experience.

The most often referred to list of Yoga's morals and ethics are those of Patanjali in his *Yoga Sūtra.* (Many other lists appear in the Yoga literature, both predating Patanjali and after him.) Remember that Patanjali's system is called Rāja Yoga, or kingly Yoga, as well as ashtanga Yoga, or eight-limbed Yoga. The eight limbs include two that address morals and ethics. They are moral "restraints" called *yama* (pronounced ya-ma), and "disciplines" called *niyama* (pronounced nee-ah-ma).[4]

---

[4] These two, yama (restraints) and niyama (disciplines), are translated in various ways by scholars. My definitions are from Eliade. One also can find the opposite translation (i.e., "discipline" for yama). Modern writers of Yoga manuals define them in different ways, such as, for yama: abstinence, conditions of behavior, attitudes toward others, and control of the mind. For niyama: self-restraint, attitudes toward ourselves, observances, and healthy practices.

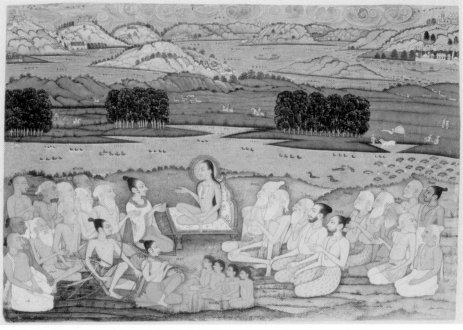

PHOTO 2.3   A yogin teaching disciples in the traditional manner in the countryside. Watercolor, c. 1757.

Yama (restraints)

1. Nonviolence *(ahimsā)*
2. Truthfulness *(satya)*
3. Nonstealing *(asteya)*
4. Continence, conserving your energy *(brahmacharya)*
5. Greedlessness *(aparigraha)*

Niyama (disciplines)

1. Purification *(saucha)*
2. Contentment *(samtosha)*
3. Austerity *(tapas)*
4. Self-study *(svādhyāya)*
5. Devotion to the Lord *(ishvara-pranidhāna)*

Yama, Restraints

The five restraints address the yogin's life in society and her relationships with other people. The practice of the restraints helps free her mind from its usual preoccupation with other people and their reactions to her.

Note: I will first describe the literal meaning of each restraint, and then the "power," called *siddhi* (pronounced sid-hee), that Patanjali says accrues to one who masters that restraint.

Nonviolence

Ahimsā (pronounced ah-him-sah´): not harming or hurting other people, animals or living things. When one lives according to ahimsā, that is, when one acts and thinks in a way that is nonharming, one gains the "power" to calm the violent feelings in others. This moral obligation is one of the justifications for vegetarianism among Hindus and yogins. It was the basis for Mahatma Gandhi's nonviolent resistance movement to the occupation of India by the British, which succeeded in gaining independence for India in 1947. Gandhi's nonviolent philosophy, and the success of his movement, inspired Dr. Martin Luther King Jr. in his fight for racial equality in the 1960s in the United States.

Truthfullness, honesty

Satya (pronounced sah-tya): thinking, speaking, and acting according to the truth as best you understand it. When one masters honesty, one obtains the "power" of having all of one's words come true. This moral precept urges us to let it be. We lie in order to change what's going to happen if the people around us know the truth. We lie to change someone's feelings about us, or to get something we want. By telling the truth, we accept the consequences of being ourselves; we accept the world we find ourselves in just as it is. We don't try to change the outcome. This takes courage, and trust in the OK-ness of the flow of life around us. This kind of acceptance, trust, and sense of OK-ness with the natural order are all prerequisites to success in Yoga, and are implied by this moral precept, truthfulness.

Nonstealing

Asteya (pronounced a-steh-ya): not taking anything that belongs to another. When one masters nonstealing, one obtains the "power" of having wealth come to one effortlessly. Nonstealing, like truthfulness, challenges us to accept our lot. If we steal, it is as if we are saying to ourselves, "The rules of the game of life aren't fair. I haven't gotten my share. So I will take what someone else has bought, earned, or worked for so that I will have my fair share." Stealing hurts others, which violates nonharming (ahimsā). But consider what stealing does *to the thief himself or herself.* If I take something that doesn't belong to me, I *act out my belief that* life isn't fair. My stealing is like a ritual or a prayer that drives the message into my brain "I am not getting my fair share." Of course stealing will never remedy the situation. It only makes it worse because one's conviction about the unfairness of life gets stronger and stronger the more one steals. This conviction prevents one from experiencing contentment. And Yoga's goal is ultimate contentment.

Continence, Conserving One's Energy, or Celibacy

Brahmacharya (pronounced brahma-chah-ri-ya): literally translates to "Godlike conduct." One who masters this precept obtains the "power" of tremendous vitality and energy. Yogins through the ages have interpreted brahmacharya in different ways. The Yoga systems that emphasize renouncing the body and its appetites, such as the Rāja Yoga of Patanjali, consider this restraint to mean celibacy and accord it a central importance in the Yoga lifestyle. Some later Yoga systems, such as Tantra Yoga and its offshoot, Hatha Yoga, don't consider celibacy to be essential or even desirable. Yogins in these systems describe brahmacharya as "conserving one's energy (not only sexual energy)," so that one can build up a reservoir of vitality for use in Yoga practices, especially meditation.

Greedlessness

Aparigraha (pronounced ah-pah-ri-grah-ha): literally, "nonreceiving," or living simply, accepting only what one really needs. One who masters greedlessness obtains the "power" of remembering one's past lives. This last sentence is a near-literal translation of the *Yoga Sūtra.* The existence of past lives is taken for granted among yogins, since the concept of reincarnation is a basic tenet of Hinduism. The yogin obtains this power of remembering past lives, because when he or she becomes free of attachment to things, to having, owning, and receiving cool stuff, even to having a body, she will see her predicament: that her clinging to things she desires keeps her stuck, bound in repeated cycles of births and rebirths. (Read more on this in Box 2.5, "Freedom, *Moksha.")* The restraint of greedlessness suggests that if we live simply, our attention and passion that is ordinarily tied up in acquiring, protecting, and worrying about our possessions will become available for more fruitful pursuits.

Niyama, Disciplines

The niyamas address the yogin's inner life, his attitudes and activities. These "disciplines" lead the yogin to states

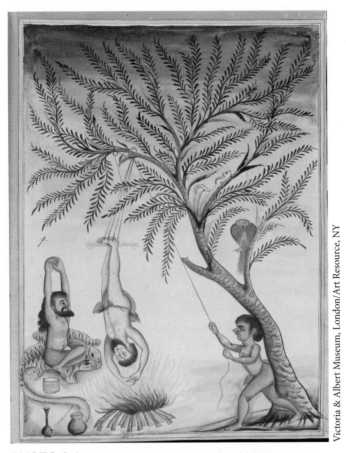

Victoria & Albert Museum, London/Art Resource, NY

PHOTO 2.4 Some yogins have assumed bizarre renunciate lifestyles to overcome their identification with their bodies. Here, an ascetic hangs over a fire as an austerity while another ascetic does a Yoga pose behind him. Painting, c. 1785.

of greater sensitivity and greater capacity to concentrate. They also orient his attention toward inner fulfillment instead of toward fulfillment of his desires.

Purification

Saucha (pronounced sow-cha): inner and outer cleanliness. One who achieves complete cleanliness, according to the *Yoga Sūtra,* becomes disinterested in one's own body and disgusted by the idea of sex with another.[5] (Note that the *Yoga Sūtra* presents a renunciate system, in contrast to Tantra Yoga's inclusive system. More on this under "Avoiding What You Want vs. Getting What You Want: Renunciation vs. Integration.)

---
[5] Vivekananda, *Rāja-Yoga,* 210.

The yogin then no longer thinks of himself as a body. He is free to discover a deeper self, undistracted by his senses. He also becomes cheerful and finds the simplest moments in his life pleasurable.

Hinduism also places a high value on cleanliness: eating clean food, keeping one's body clean, and keeping one's home clean. In Yoga (especially Hatha Yoga) this is taken further to imply a super-clean inner state that results from removing impurities and obstructions in one's body by the practice of a variety of yogic techniques. Two purification practices common to most Yoga systems are a "cleansing" diet and fasting (abstaining from food completely for a number of days).

Contentment

Samtosha (pronounced sum-tow-sha): calmness, peacefulness, and quietude. One who achieves contentment obtains the "power" of feeling inner bliss, the happiness that naturally comes from simply being alive and aware. This niyama, like the restraint of greedlessness, directs the yogin toward a simple, uncluttered life. Like cleanliness, this frees the yogin's mind so it can become quiet, a prerequisite for overcoming one's limited self-image.

Austerity

Tapas (pronounced tah-pahs): disciplines that require willpower or require one to tolerate discomfort. An example of tolerating discomfort is when you continue to sit motionless even when you feel agitated. By mastering austerities, the yogin attains a state of purity, and attains a "power" of heightened sensing, such that she is able to see and hear things that are usually beyond the capacities of an ordinary person's senses. Many Yoga systems agree that excessive austerities are unhelpful, and warn against them. However, throughout Yoga's history a number of influential

BOX **2.2**

Avoiding What You Want vs. Getting What You Want: Renunciation vs. Integration

If these moral precepts are starting to sound to you like guidelines for monks and nuns, you are right. The yogin described by Patanjali in the *Yoga Sūtra* is a renunciate, who turns away from the world and its pleasures and entanglements. Later Yoga systems such as Hatha Yoga, which incorporate these same moral precepts, usually interpret them differently, as in the case of celibacy (brahmacharya), mentioned earlier. Another example: contentment (samtosha) for a renunciate might be an ultra-simple life in a Yoga monastery. For a Tantra yogin it could be spending a few hours a day doing Yoga practices, or taking a quiet walk, or sitting alone by a river. In contrast to renunciate Yoga, the Yoga systems that include one's involvement in life's pleasures are called "integrative Yoga."

schools have used extreme austerities to "burn up" (another translation of tapas) the yogin's attachments or to break the yogin's mind's trance with body identification and sensual desires. Some examples of these extreme austerities are going without food for several weeks, sitting outside in winter for a whole day with only a loincloth on, or remaining in a painful posture for an hour. (See the box "Avoiding What You Want vs. Getting What You Want.")

Hatha Yoga utilizes austerities (of the moderate sort) as a way to refine one's mind and to awaken a clearer view of reality and who one is. Hatha Yoga's austerities take the form of the multitude of practices: moving or posing one's body, slowing down one's breathing, concentrating one's attention on one thing for a long time, and so on. (More on this in Chapter 3.)

Self-Study

Svādhyāya (pronounced swah'-dhi-yah'-ya): investigating one's mind, inquiring into its nature and thereby discovering the eternal wisdom, the divine in oneself. This niyama is often translated as "study of the scriptures."

Feuerstein states this elegantly: "The purpose of svādhyāya is not intellectual learning; it is absorption into ancient wisdom. It is the meditative pondering of truths revealed by seers and sages who have traversed those remote regions where the mind cannot follow and only the heart receives and is changed.[6]

Devotion to the Lord

Ishvara-pranidhāna (pronounced eesh-wa-ra prah-ni-dha'-nah): surrendering to the divine being within you, to your highest self. By mastering divine surrender the yogin attains the highest state of understanding. This discipline is the most controversial of the five, because in most ways Patanjali's system and most other Yoga systems aren't God-centered. Many Yoga schools don't include the idea of God at all. In Jnana Yoga, the highest reality is called the Self, parama-ātman. Nonetheless, Patanjali clearly identifies the Lord, *ishvara,* as an essential part of the yogin's inner journey toward spiritual awareness. One modern writer, James Hewitt, was clearly uncomfortable

---

[6] Feuerstein, *The Yoga Tradition,* 247.

The "Yoga of Action," Kriya Yoga

Patanjali writes in the *Yoga Sūtra* that the practice of three of the five niyamas (austerity [tapas], self-study [swādhyāya], and devotion to the Lord [ishvara-pranidhāna]) is called Kriya Yoga (pronounced kree-yah). Patanjali is more famous for his other Yoga: the eight-fold path, ashtanga Yoga, or Rāja Yoga. (See Box 1.12, "The Eight Limbs of Rāja Yoga".) Feuerstein suggests that Kriya Yoga, however, was Patanjali's greater contribution to the Yoga legacy. He writes, "Even though Patanjali's Yoga has achieved fame for its eightfold path, it is likely that this particular systematization was merely cited by Patanjali and that his own contribution to Yoga was Kriya-Yoga.[9]

In recent times the term *Kriya Yoga* has come to refer to the Yoga system taught by the renowned yogi Paramahansa Yogananda (1893–1952),and by the mythical guru who preceded Yogananda by several generations, Babaji. This Yoga system combines elements of Hatha Yoga and Bhakti Yoga.

with the inclusion of God or Lord in the "disciplines." He says, "Ishvara, the Supreme Being, is probably a later interpolation into Patanjali's *Yoga Sūtras,* in which he sits uneasily as a model (of pure spirit). . . ."[7]

The Yoga systems before Patanjali (pre-classical Yoga) and after him (post-classical Yoga) view God, if they include God at all, as the Supreme Reality of which everything is an expression. An analogy for this that I used earlier is the ocean water appearing for a time as a wave. But the wave *really* is water *taking form* as a wave. It is not separate from the water of which it is made. This is called *a nondual* philosophy, whereas Patanjali's philosophy is *dualistic,* contrasting starkly with these other Yoga systems.[8] Patanjali paints a picture of a Lord or God that is eternally *separate from* human life and nature. Patanjali envisions the awakened state of consciousness as overcoming one's nature, one's body, emotions, thoughts, and so on, and identifying with a spiritual Self (purusha, pronounced poo-roo-sha) that stands apart from nature.

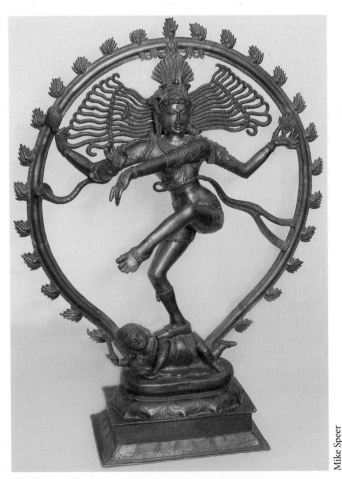

Mike Speer

PHOTO 2.5   Many Yoga schools don't include the idea of God at all. This statue depicts the god Shiva.

---

[7] Hewitt, *The Complete Yoga Book,* 420. also see Eliade, *Patanjali and yoga,* 88.

[8] Feuerstein, *The Yoga Tradition,* 248.

[9] Feuerstein, *The Shambhala Encyclopedia of Yoga,* 159.

in solitude, scant diet, fasting, silence, noncontact, and indifference.[10]

Completing the Journey to One's True Self

I stated at the opening of this chapter that the reason few people have experienced their big "S" Self, their ātman, is because it is not easy to do. Consciousness, which is our camera through which we perceive ourselves, gets stuck easily. Yoga is a method of getting unstuck. One of Yoga's methods, we learned, is to *train for* the big unsticking event, when the light goes on and we figuratively wake up. Some Yoga boot camps were pretty austere. These are the renunciate varieties of Yoga, the kind that urge the yogin to withdraw from the world. These Yoga schools were dominant for most of Yoga's history. In about the first half of the first millennium CE, as you learned in Chapter 1, Tantra Yoga emerged as an alternative to the renunciate Yoga schools such as Jnana Yoga (also called Vedanta) and Rāja Yoga (also see Box 2.4). Tantra Yoga spawned Hatha Yoga, which retained Tantra's inclusive or integrative philosophy. Hatha Yoga developed into the modern exercise Yoga systems that I call Āsana Yoga. The modern systems retain some of Hatha Yoga and Tantra Yoga's philosophy, especially their inclusiveness and their attention to body-conditioning.

Tantra Yoga's philosophy of body inclusion made yogic spirituality more attainable for the common family person in India,[11] and it has made Yoga practice more accessible and relevant to modern college students in North America. In short, you can buy cool stuff, enjoy a fine meal, hang out

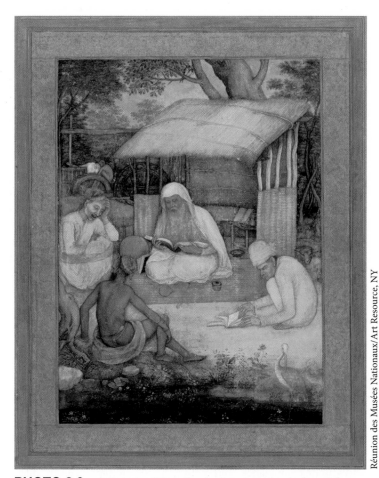

PHOTO 2.6 Artists traditionally depicted yogins in forest (or other rural) settings, indicating their renunciation of ordinary society, as shown in this 13th-century painting.

Réunion des Musées Nationaux/Art Resource, NY

Other Lists of Yoga's Ethics and Morals

The list of ten morals and ethics described above is from the *Yoga Sūtra* (100–200 CE), and it is by far the most quoted list of Yoga ethics. Many other lists exist in the Yoga literature, often, as in the *Yoga Sūtra,* called yama and niyama. As alluded to in our discussion of the discipline "devotion to the Lord," some of the lists exclude any mention of God or Lord and view the divine in a nondual form. Some other lists include even more religious references than those in the *Yoga Sūtra,* such as the *Uddhava-Gita,* which includes faith *(shradha),* worship *(arcane),* and pilgrimage *(tirtha-atana).* Some Yoga systems are more renunciate than was Pantajali's, and so list restraints or disciplines such as living

---

[10] Ibid., 204, 340.

[11] Danielou, *Gods of Love and Ecstasy,* 15-16; Feuerstein, *Yoga Tradition,* 343.

A Note about the Varieties of Yoga Exploration

I state that the renunciate varieties of Yoga, which include Jnana and Rāja Yoga, require the yogin to withdraw from ordinary human society. This isn't completely accurate, because there are and have always been so many different sects of yogins within any of the Yoga schools. India is a land of incessant experimentation with states of consciousness. The history of Yoga is full of stories of rebellious yogins who try new methods that violate the dogma of the day and irritate the religious elite. Many schools in every era have spawned their antithesis. Here is an example: the great modern Jnana yogin, Ramana Maharshi (1879–1950), taught that anyone in any situation, renunciate or worldly, could realize the Self by inquiring, "Who am I?"

Here's another example: some Tantra yogins have assumed bizarre renunciate lifestyles to overcome their identification with their bodies and their sense pleasures, such as living in the cremation grounds and meditating, covered in ash, while sitting on the burnt remains of a human body.

My generalizations about renunciate Yoga systems and inclusive or integrative Yoga systems apply especially to the philosophies of the major Yoga schools as evidenced in the Yoga literature.

with the gang in the student union, and still be on a viable Yoga path. According to Tantra philosophy, your appetites, your sensations, and even your thoughts are all just movements of the divine, all just movements of your Self-that-is-also-everything. All of these— appetites, sensations, thoughts—can be followed to their source, to the Absolute, to Brahman.

Don't misunderstand. Tantra does not say, "Do whatever you please." Traditional Tantra prescribes a rigorous, challenging lifestyle. It includes moral and ethical behavior (yama and niyama), just as do all Yoga systems.

How does Tantra Yoga teach a person to follow her sensations and thoughts to the "source"? Tantra teaches an extensive curriculum of *preparatory* practices that purify and strengthen the yogin. And it teaches a variety of more *advanced practices* that induce peak states of awareness. These body/mind practices involve power sounds (mantra), visualization (yantra, pronounced yahn-tra),

breath control (prānāyāma), and ultimately, deep meditation.

Conditioning and Habits

Let's look at Yoga's philosophy of human habits and liberation from habits, for in it we will see a number of elements that appear in the philosophy of modern Yoga lineages.

To attain maximum awareness, the yogin must overcome his tendency to live today just as he did yesterday. All his experiences, all his thoughts, all his actions have left an impression in him. These impressions are called *samskāra* (pronounced sahm-skah´-rah) by Patanjali in the *Yoga Sūtra*. Samskāra literally translates to "activators" or habits. Most of the yogin's past impressions, samskāras, reinforce his ego identification, his fixed idea of who he is and the sort of world he lives in. In other words, the yogin's past experience creates his habits of mind and thought.

Here's the mess we are in, according to Yoga philosophy: because we have felt pleasure and pain before, and those experiences have left us with habits, we try to continually re-create pleasant events and re-avoid unpleasant ones. This is, of course, natural and healthy but becomes problematic when we spend *all* of our mental and physical energy on this task; it's problematic when we believe that we can actually find *true happiness and fulfillment* chasing after that which we desire. Happiness is forever elusive for the person caught in attachment and rejection because getting a new computer doesn't remove your desire for new shoes or for an even more powerful computer after a while.

The Dawning of Wisdom

Yoga offers two different ways out of this perpetual mess: rise above it all or experience it. Rising above it is renunciation, and involves suppressing your thoughts and impulses and replacing them with a one-pointed focus on something, such as your breath or the Divine. Experiencing it means feeling your wants, your anger, your dislikes, your sadness, your frustration, and your joy—in short, using your refined awareness to accept yourself and to relax to such a point that you see that *you are* that which you seek: pure bliss and ultimate peace.

According to Tantra philosophy you grow wise about your *wanting* of some experiences and your *rejection* of others by developing the power of your mind to focus, so you can focus on your experience *now*. Then you may recognize your cravings and dislikes as activities of your conditioned mind, the trajectory into your present experience of events that have happened to you in the past. You may become suspicious of your conviction that by attaining the things you desire and ridding yourself of the things you

dislike that you will be happy. This growing wisdom about your want-filled thoughts and your rejection-filled thoughts will make you less preoccupied with these thoughts and will free up your mental space and your field of awareness so that you can focus on your here-and-now experience: your clothes touching your skin, your breath in your nostrils, your hands holding this book. Focusing on your here-and-now experience quiets your constant mental chatter and shows you, perhaps briefly, a reality that is bigger, brighter, and richer than your familiar one. Focusing your attention with potency gained from practice can part the veil of your stuck-ness and reveal . . . you, the unconditioned, spectacular you (see Box 2.5).

This process may sound entirely self-absorbing, and therefore selfish. What about other people? In fact, when we work on our own self-awareness as prescribed by Yoga, we naturally become more concerned about the well-being of others, both human and animal. As we improve our own state of contentment, we become more valuable to those around us: we are more inclined to help others, and we are better able to help because we have more insight and more energy.

Applying Tantra Yoga Philosophy

The traditional yogin sees that a pursuit of happiness and contentment that requires her *image* to change, her *idea* of who she is to change, is doomed to fail. Here's how that works: she feels, let's say, unhappy with her looks, and with her grades compared to her friends' grades, and with her style of conversation around guys (she can't think of anything "funny" to say). So she vows to change: to get better grades, to change her hairstyle, and to be more relaxed with guys. If she can succeed

Freedom, Moksha

Just as the yogin can loosen the cords of conditioning, of samskāra, and just as she can loosen the cords of I-ness, she can, in the final loosening, lose the need to be reborn in a human body after her body dies. This is a teaching common to all Yoga traditions. "Freedom," *moksha* (pronounced moke-shah), is a natural extension of the philosophy of realized ecstasy, samādhi.

According to this theory, our self-building actions, those that are impelled by our conditioning, our samskāras, create repercussions in the future that eventually will come to fruition. This is called "the law of causality," or *karma* (pronounced kahr-mah). Our karma, the residue from our actions, from this lifetime and from our previous lifetimes, creates our present circumstances. As long as we act with an I-bound or ego-bound consciousness, we create more karma, more waves of "cause" that ripple into the future, kind of like bad luck. These waves cause us to be born over and over again in human bodies so that we can live out the effects of our karma and learn from our experience.

The theory of karma teaches that if we can overcome our conditioning and become our true Selves, we no longer act with any self-interest. We don't have preferences for pleasure, comfort, or happiness. Our "I," who might "have happiness" isn't there. Such a person thinks, feels, moves as the Supreme, as the parama-ātman, the Self that is the Self of all. The actions of the Supreme don't create karma, so a person who is identified with the Supreme, who is enlightened, as this state is called, isn't creating any more karma. She isn't reborn after she dies. She attains freedom, moksha. This is the ultimate goal of all traditional Yoga practice.

at these efforts, she will feel better about herself, she thinks. If she can't, she will renew her resolve to change, or give up and feel terrible about herself.

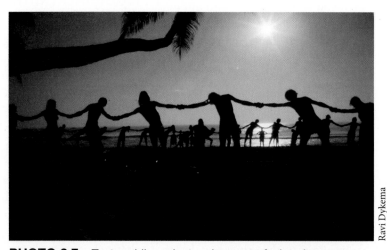

PHOTO 2.7   Tantra philosophy teaches us to feel and accept our here-and-now experience, whether it is pleasant or unpleasant.

Ravi Dykema

But even if she succeeds in changing, she will feel OK only briefly. After a short while, she will reset her standards of prettiness, academic excellence, and chattiness and find herself lacking. Over and over again this will happen. She will think she's deficient in important ways, she will feel bad about herself, and she will try hard to fix herself by changing how she acts or looks, so others will see her differently and she can then revise her own assessment of her OK-ness. In reality, according to Yoga philosophy, she's perfect already (as you have read before, she is the absolute, Brahman). Her feeling of deficiency is an illusion, a trick of her mind. Her OK-ness and attractiveness are natural ever-present qualities she can never lose. Her mind (and all minds) can always come up with images of *more* OK people and *more* attractive people. (By the way, her mind can also always find less-OK people with whom to compare herself.)

Yoga's solution to this conundrum is for her to turn off her crazy mind and find that perfection that just *is* always present. The way Yoga prescribes that she feel her intrinsic perfection and OK-ness is to bring her attention and senses to *this moment,* to her immediate experiences. Yoga prescribes that she feel her feet pressing into the floor, that she feel her breath moving deeply in and out, that she feel her arms and hands reaching out beside her. This focus will quiet her mind and awaken in her feelings of pleasure, of calm, of OK-ness, and of beauty. These supportive feelings won't depend on what other people think about her clothes that day. These feelings will also be available again and again when she quiets her mind and tunes in to her sensations. She might get good at this focusing even when she isn't doing Yoga, although she might find that a regular Yoga practice helps her tune in to herself and helps her interrupt her run-on thoughts, many of which are paranoid (such as, "Did my comment about class sound stupid?").

Lots of people don't think this kind of fullness exists inside them. They think they can only get it from their performance, from the images other people hold in their minds about them and the images they hold in their own minds about themselves.

In answer to these doubters, Yoga philosophy says, in a way, "Try Yoga, and see what happens. See if you feel more at home in your body and mind. Don't believe it just because someone wrote it down somewhere. Do the practice and see what happens."

3

Hatha Yoga, the Yoga of Balanced Energy

This book focuses mainly on Hatha (pronounced hut-ha) Yoga and its modern offshoots, the exercise-oriented systems of Yoga. Hatha Yoga is the primary parent of most modern Yoga teachings around the world. Along with Tantra Yoga (Tantrism), Hatha Yoga teaches the wide variety of body positions or poses called āsanas, which are the most common element in modern Yoga. In fact, most people think of Yoga as exclusively an āsana system, a physical system, similar to weight training or aerobics.[1] You now know that Yoga is much more. In this chapter we'll investigate the theories and practices of "traditional Hatha Yoga" as represented by Yoga lineages that teach most or all of the practices listed or described in the old literature of Hatha Yoga, especially the *Goraksha-Samhitā*, the *Hatha-Yoga-Pradīpikā*, the *Gheranda-Samhitā*, and the *Shiva-Samhitā*. Through studying traditional Hatha Yoga, we can understand how modern "daughter" Yoga systems draw from, and expand on, the Hatha Yoga tradition.

---

[1] In fact, one author says that there *is* a traditional Yoga system that is only concerned with the "training of the physical body as an end in itself," called Ghatastha Yoga. Bernard, *Hatha Yoga*, 16.

Overview of the Theory of Hatha Yoga

The Feuerstein quote in Box 3.1 alludes to the goal of Hatha Yoga, which is "spiritual perfection." But for a Yoga practitioner whose experience falls short of "perfection" or "enlightenment," Hatha practices can still be most helpful. They can improve the yogin's mental clarity, powers of concentration, energy levels, physical comfort, and they can calm anxiety.

According to Yoga theory, these practices work in large part by producing a change in the yogin's *energy body,* which in turn creates a change in the physical body.

Hatha Yoga practices produce these results by

- Cleansing and purifying the organs, muscles, and energy body
- Strengthening, stretching, and relaxing the muscles and joints
- Improving the ability to balance
- Regulating the breath, and increasing the capacity for breath
- Focusing the mind on sounds *(nada)*, images *(yantra)*, and especially sensations in specific places *(desha)* to the exclusion of all else

Scholars and Sages on Hatha Yoga

In Tantrism [and Hatha Yoga], the human body acquires an importance it had never before attained in the spiritual history of India. . . . The Upanishadic and post-Upanishadic pessimism and asceticism are swept away. The body is no longer the source of pain, but the most reliable and effective instrument at man's disposal for "conquering death." [This can be interpreted as achieving freedom, moksha; see Chapter 2.] And since liberation can be gained even in this life, the body must be preserved as long as possible, and in perfect condition, precisely as an aid to meditation.

—Mircea Eliade [2]

It was the adepts of Tantrism [and Hatha Yoga] . . . who inaugurated a new attitude toward the human body and bodily existence in general. In pre-Tantric times, the body was often looked upon, in Gnostic fashion, as a source of defilement, as the enemy of the spirit. . . . What Tantric masters aspired to was to create a transubstantiated body, which they called "adamantine" (vajra) or "divine" (daiva)—a body not made of flesh but of immortal substance, of Light. Instead of regarding the body as a meat tube doomed to fall prey to sickness and death, they viewed it as a dwelling place of the Divine, and as the cauldron for accomplishing spiritual perfection. For them, enlightenment was a whole-body event.

—Georg Feuerstein [3]

Just as rock salt [is dissolved] in water, so the Absolute extends to the body [of the enlightened yogin].

—The Yoga-Shikha-Upanishad (1.163), translated by Feuerstein [4]

- Relaxing to the point of losing one's sense of having a body
- Emptying the mind so no thoughts (or few thoughts) arise

All of these practices achieve their results by creating changes in the yogin's energy body.

The Energy Body and the Five Bodies

Hatha Yoga teaches that we each have a physical body as well as other "bodies" that are not physical, that is, not made of atoms and molecules. These other bodies are considered to be made of "energy," somewhat like the electrical energy by which your nervous system functions. That is why I translate Hatha Yoga as the "Yoga of balanced energy." This idea of a nonphysical body is shared by most other spiritual traditions. Parallel traditions around the world suggest that life, consciousness, and spirit manifest in a person in more than his or her physical body.

The most common model of energy bodies in Yoga is the theory of the "five sheaths" (pancha-kosha, pronounced pan-cha ko-sha), or five bodies, first described in the *Taittiriya-Upanishad* (ninth century BCE) and discussed thereafter in many other works.

The five bodies (pancha-kosha) are:

1. The "body composed of food" (*anna-maya-kosha*), the physical body.

---

[2] Eliade, *Yoga: Immortality and Freedom*, 227.

[3] Feuerstein, *The Yoga Tradition*, 382.

[4] Ibid., 382.

2. The "body composed of life force" (*prāna-maya-kosha*), sometimes called the emotional body or the body of breath. This is the body that contains channels through which the energy, *prāna*, flows. These channels are called *nādīs* (pronounced nah-dees).

3. The "body composed of mind" (*mano-maya-kosha*), the intellect.

4. The "body composed of awareness" (*vijñāna-maya-kosha*), also called the body of understanding or wisdom.

5. The "body composed of bliss" (*ānanda-maya-kosha*), the body through which one experiences the Absolute, the ultimate Truth, which is said to be intensely blissful (*ānanda*).[5]

The body that is the easiest to feel and to influence, other than your physical body, is your body of prāna, also called the emotional body, or body of breath. Hatha Yoga emphasizes breath awareness and breath control because altering your breathing pattern is the most potent way for you to affect your energy bodies. Please explore this by trying the exercise in Box 3.2.

When your energy body changes, your physical body changes and your perception changes. So Hatha Yoga practices represent a kind of holistic fitness regimen for your consciousness and your instrument of perception. Hatha Yoga seeks to clarify your view, your perception of reality, to such an extent that you can't help but see the whole picture, the fundamental reality that is always present.

You can think of your perception as a spotlight, like the one that shines on the singer at a rock concert. Hatha Yoga practice *brightens* your perception spotlight, so you can see more detail, more depth, and more subtlety. And Hatha Yoga trains you to *aim* your spotlight of perception so you can keep it on one thing, whatever you choose, longer. These two tools, *clarity* and *control*, are essential to Hatha Yoga.

Clarity

Hatha Yoga works on clarity of perception by teaching an elaborate program of purification and cleansing practices. The *Hatha-Yoga-Pradīpikā* and *Gheranda-Samhitā* call one set of these practices the "six acts," or *shatkarma* (pronounced shaht kar-mah). These practices work on removing impurities and obstructions from your nasal passages, your sinuses, your bronchial tubes, your lungs, your digestive organs, and your circulatory system. Hatha Yoga's cleansing regime also works on your more subtle "bodies," like your nervous system, your emotional body and your mind. These cleansing procedures include personal hygiene techniques like the nasal cleanser taught in Box 3.3, breathing practices, body positions and

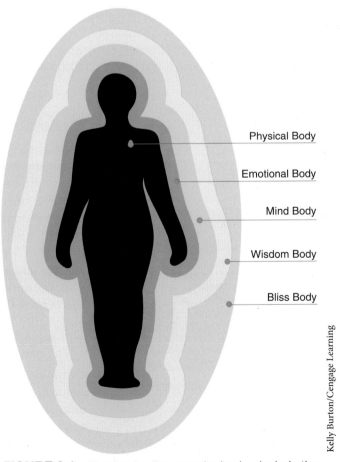

Physical Body

Emotional Body

Mind Body

Wisdom Body

Bliss Body

Kelly Burton/Cengage Learning

FIGURE 3.1 The five bodies, pancha kosha, include the physical body and four energy bodies.

[5] Feuerstein, *The Shambhala Encyclopedia of Yoga*, 157; Feuerstein, *The Yoga Tradition*, 132.

BOX 3.2

Feeling Your Energy Body

Try this exercise. Sit comfortably with both feet flat on the floor and your back erect, not leaning back in your chair. Notice for a minute how you feel, and how your body feels. Now close your eyes and take ten deep, slow, easy breaths, feeling your chest and belly move as you breathe. After you are done, notice how you feel again. Do you feel more tense or more relaxed? How calm or agitated do you feel?

BOX 3.3

A Purification Practice

One purification practice of Hatha Yoga that anyone can do is called "water cleansing" (jala-neti, pronounced jah-la ne-tee). Fill a cup half full with body-temperature water. Shake non-iodized salt into it and stir until it tastes similar to your tears or to sea water. Hold one nostril closed. Submerge your other nostril in the water with your head tipped to the side and suck gently, in short sniffs, perhaps five times, until water comes out your mouth [3.1]. This feels just like getting water in your nose when you are swimming in the ocean. Then do the same with the other nostril. Don't blow your nose right after doing this, as this can force liquid into your eustachian tubes that pass into your middle ears, which can cause an ear infection. You can gently exhale water from both nostrils at once into the sink. Don't close one nostril while you blow through the other. Water cleansing clears your nose, sinuses, and throat, and is traditionally used as a preparation for Yoga breathing practices.

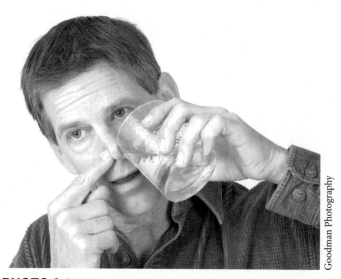

PHOTO 3.1   Cleaning your nostrils with salt water is a cleansing exercise called *neti*.

Goodman Photography

Control

We learned that Hatha Yoga trains you to aim your spotlight of perception so you can keep it on one thing, whatever you choose, longer. This is mental control. Mental control is concentration. (Please try the exercise in Box 3.4.) Here is an example of a way you already often use this skill. You are able to pay attention to a lecturer in the front of the classroom instead of to your classmates' conversation three seats away from you because of your power of concentration. This power, this ability to concentrate, can be strengthened by using it more, the way you strengthen a muscle by using it. Many Hatha Yoga practices require concentration. Every practice that involves the body, for example, requires that you

movements, mental exercises (such as visualizing pure water flowing through you), and dietary guidelines.

BOX 3.4

A Concentration Exercise

A Hatha Yoga concentration exercise that you might try is called "vital energy focus" (prāna dhāranā): sit with your back straight, not leaning back in your chair, or sit cross-legged on a carpeted floor [3.3]. Close your eyes and focus your attention on your abdomen moving as you breathe. Feel it puffing out slightly as you breathe in, and feel it drawing in slightly as you breathe out. Keep feeling your belly like this, while you relax the rest of you. Let your thoughts come and go. Just keep feeling your belly moving. If you find at some point that your attention is no longer on your abdomen, bring your focus there again. It is OK if you need to bring your awareness back to your belly over and over. Keep doing this for fifteen minutes.

If you practice this exercise regularly for a month, you will likely succeed at extending your ability to focus on your breath without your mind wandering. A full minute is quite an accomplishment. Five minutes of sustained concentration would indicate that you have substantial skill in dhāranā, yogic concentration. An advanced yogin should be able to hold her mind on a single focus point for half an hour.

focus on your sensations, that you feel deeply what happens in your muscles, joints, and breathing as you move. This kind of focusing is concentration, also called one-pointed awareness, or *dhāranā*.[6] (Remember,

this is one of the limbs of "eight-limbed Yoga," *ashtanga Yoga*, or *Rāja Yoga*. See Box 1.12, "The Eight Limbs of Rāja Yoga".) Theos Bernard writes about this control and about the role of poses (āsana) in Hatha Yoga in general:

> There is not a single āsana that is not intended directly or indirectly to quiet the mind; however, for the advanced meditation practices of Yoga there are only two postures that are considered essential. These are siddhāsana and padmāsana [each are cross-legged sitting poses]. The other āsanas have been devised to build up different parts of the body and to develop the needed strength that is required by the rigid physical disciplines imposed upon the student. The teacher emphasizes that the primary purpose of the āsanas is the reconditioning of the system, both mind and body, so as to effect the highest possible standard of muscular tone, mental health and organic vigor.[7]

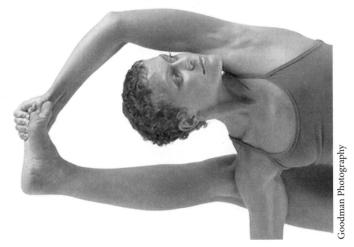

PHOTO 3.2   Yoga poses develop tremendous strength along with powers of concentration.

Goodman Photography

---

[6] Eliade writes, "It goes without saying that [one-pointed awareness] can be obtained only through the practice of numerous exercises and techniques, in which physiology plays a role of primary importance. One cannot obtain one-pointedness if, for example, the body is in a tiring or uncomfortable posture, or if the respiration is disorganized, unrhythmical." *Yoga, Immortality, and Freedom*, 48.

---

[7] Bernard, *Hatha Yoga*, 25.

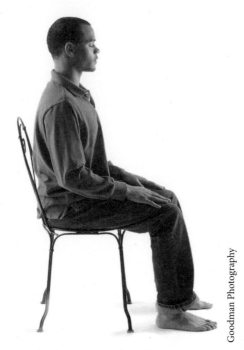

Goodman Photography

PHOTO 3.3 Focus your attention on your abdomen as you breathe. Feel it puffing out slightly as you breathe in, and feel it drawing in slightly as you breathe out.

Although poses (āsanas) are the most widely known practice of Hatha Yoga, another bodily practice is more central to the task of controlling the mind in concentration. That practice is breath control (*pranāyāma,* which derives from *prāna* = vital energy + *āyāma* = extension or control).

The *Hatha Yoga Pradīpikā* states, "When prāna (the life force) moves, the mind also moves. When prāna ceases to move, the mind becomes motionless. . . . Therefore, one should control prāna." [8]

This formula, "quieting the breath quiets the mind," or, more literally, "stopping the breath stops the mind," is found in all the main Hatha Yoga texts. "Stopping the breath" means holding the breath for some seconds with each cycle of breathing. For example, breathing in for six seconds, holding in for six seconds, and exhaling for six seconds. Also found in all the main texts of Hatha Yoga is the requirement that the yogin prepare for breath control, pranāyāma, by first completing the cleansing and purification of his body and "energy channels" (nādīs),[9] discussed earlier. (For more on nādīs, see the section "The Energy Body and the Five Bodies" earlier in this chapter.)

Control of your mind is made more possible by controlling your body: your muscles, your movements, and your breath. An advanced student wrote in an assigned paper about her experience with breath (pranāyāma):

Just like last semester I found complete comfort in the held-out breath. It is at this time when I feel most alive, yet most relaxed. I feel like I sink to levels of relaxation

unattainable without it. I remember my thought the first time we did it this semester was, "I'm home." Every part of me inside and out melts away. Subtly it washes away layers of veils and brings me to a place of absolute quiet. The wonderful thing about it is that it is *nothing* [her italics]. There are no fireworks or unreal feelings, the state I experience is pure being and that is it. . . . Because this experience was so unexpected I think maybe I was more open than I would have been if I had been waiting for something to happen. That's just the thing, nothing happened, everything *stopped* happening. It was beautiful! [10]

Surrender, Letting Go

Control of your mind has two parts: controlling and letting go. You don't have the kind of control that Hatha Yoga aims at until you can relax your effort as well as engage it. This definition of control is clearer when we think of muscular control. To bend your arm you must *contract* your bicep muscle. To straighten it you must *relax* your bicep muscle. If you hold your bicep in a contraction all the time, you can't use your arm very well. If you hold your mind in an effortful mode all the time, even in one-pointed awareness, you can't use your mind very well, either.

Letting go means not doing, not striving, not pursuing a goal, not trying. At the mental level, when meditation (dhyāna) becomes effortless it is called "ecstasy" (samādhi). The person who concentrates to the point of attaining Yoga meditation and then samādhi loses his sense of "I am meditating" because his sense of being a doer dissolves. Eliade alludes

---

[8] Ibid., 54, from *Hatha Yoga Pradīpikā,* ii, 2.
[9] Ibid.

[10] Student paper for Yoga II at Naropa University.

to this when he writes, "They, [concentration, meditation, and ecstasy] are so much alike that the yogin who attempts one of them (concentration, for example) cannot easily remain in it, and sometimes finds himself, *quite against his will,* slipping over into meditation or [samādhi, ecstasy]" (my italics).[11]

Another way to understand the mental letting go of Yoga is for us to revisit Yoga philosophy, which says that your "self" is really the Absolute (Brahman), but mistakenly thinks it is separate and unique. People get stuck, contracted around the image of themselves as a separate individual. The task of all Yoga, then, is to unstick you, to uncontract you, so you can realize your splendorous Real Self, which just is, and which isn't propped up by ideas or reinforced by thoughts. After the yogin purifies his body, develops breath control that leads to mental concentration, and sustains that concentration in an unbroken flow (meditation) he has gone as far as he can with his own effort. His next challenge is to let go enough to dissolve, expand, explode, surrender, and *relax* into true being, into true Self awareness, ecstasy. George Feuerstein eloquently expresses this idea:

> Relaxation is the alpha and omega of Yoga. How so? According to the yogic worldview, ordinary life, revolving around the accumulation of pleasurable and painful experiences, is a result of the contraction of consciousness. In its pure state, as the transcendental Self, consciousness is completely unrestricted and free. However, through wrongful identification with a particular body-mind, the spacious consciousness of the Self seemingly contracts to create the limited awareness of the psyche (jiva). In

truth, the Self never contracts at all. The illusion of contraction is the problem. Yoga therefore seeks to undermine this illusion by which all unenlightened beings bind themselves. It endeavors to systematically remove all those binds that help maintain the illusion. This endeavor can be viewed as an extensive process of disentanglement, or purification, or relaxation.

In this broader sense, relaxation denotes letting go of the tension that creates the illusion of the ego's individuality and separateness. Thus relaxation is not merely relaxation of the body but also of the mind—our opinions, concerns, hopes, and attitudes. It is the master key to all levels of the yogic enterprise. But for most people, bodily relaxation is an excellent starting point for this more comprehensive process of letting go.[12]

"Letting Go" in the Practice of Yoga Poses and Yoga Breathing

Bodily relaxation involves exploring how one might perform a backbending pose with less effort. Can you, for example, relax your face more, or your shoulders, while still using other muscles to do the pose? I call this "not doing in the middle of doing." Another way of achieving this kind of relaxation-in-the-midst-of-activity is to do your Yoga poses in such a way that you would get a C grade for effort if someone could feel inside you and grade you. This means backing off from full effort. To experience this, do a Yoga position first with full effort, trying for your idea of perfection, really going for it. Then reduce your effort a little while you keep moving or holding the pose. Notice that you feel a bit more sensation in your body. And your breath is

---

[11] Eliade, *Yoga: Immortality, and Freedom,* 70.

[12] Feuerstein, *The Shambhala Guide to Yoga,* 51.

deeper, easier. Your energy is flowing more strongly at this time. Excess tension blocks energy flow and sensation, whereas the appropriate amount of effort and tension increases energy and sensation. This theory of Hatha Yoga[13] has some far-reaching implications.

Here is a scenario that illustrates the theory of tension that reduces feelings and sensation: when you feel really happy all of a sudden, full of joy, you may react to your feeling in a curious way. You may react by tensing up a little and constraining your movements and your voice because you are afraid you might appear weird or stupid, or in some way unlike your usual self. You might do the same when you feel really angry. For most people this reaction to a feeling is unconscious. They aren't aware of tensing up. Your social situation may indeed require of you that you hide or reduce your feelings. But here's another way to understand what is happening here: You can't tolerate the intensity of your feeling; it is like too much voltage in a wire, so you shut it off by tensing up. You instinctively know how to turn down the energy volume; your body knows how to tense muscles to reduce feelings.

This is perfectly appropriate sometimes. Yet, other times, you may *want* to feel really happy and show it, or mad and show it. If you become aware of what you do in your body when you turn off the feeling, you can choose to relax instead, and let your feelings rush through you.

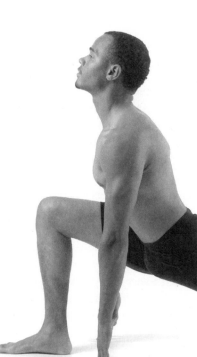

Goodman Photography

PHOTO 3.4   When you relax your effort a little while holding a pose, notice that you feel more sensations and your breath is deeper and easier. In contrast, excess tension blocks breathing and sensation.

---

[13] Eliade writes, "The important thing is that *āsana* gives the body a stable rigidity, at the same time reducing physical effort to a minimum. Thus, one avoids the irritating feeling of fatigue, of enervation [reduction of energy] in certain parts of the body, one regulates the physical processes, and so allows the attention to devote itself solely to the fluid part of consciousness . . . effort must disappear, the position of meditation must become natural; only then does it further concentration." *Yoga: Immortality, and Freedom,* 53.

The skill of "doing/not doing" or "getting a *C* for effort" can help you be more comfortable and poised in stressful or intense situations. My students have reported that this does indeed happen.

A student wrote in a class paper:

When I am in that hell place, if I can practice Yoga to become aware of the sensations in my body, give it space, and treat it with kindness, something entirely different happens. Things become OK. I am more able to accept that it's there and suddenly it doesn't feel quite so painful any more. The rough edges come down, my world relaxes a bit, and after some time the experience usually does subside. And not by avoiding it, but because I have given it space in my body through yoga, and accepted it there. Yoga is like the key out of my neurotic prison.[14]

The Anatomy of Awakening: Kundalinī and Chakras

The practices and energy states to which I will be alluding in this section are rarely taught in modern Yoga classes, and then only to advanced yogins in certain Yoga lineages. I mention them here because they were once a central component of Hatha Yoga practice. No student of Hatha Yoga who reads scholarly works or translations of Sanskrit classics could miss the numerous mentions of exotic energies and the subtle body transformations they induce, notably the *kundalinī* energy (pronounced koon-duh-lin-ee, a powerful body energy) and the *chakras* (pronounced

---

[14] Student paper tor Yoga I at Naropa University.

chah-krah, literally "wheels," or subtle energy centers in your body). See Box 3.5.

I deduce from my reading of the literature that during Hatha Yoga's heyday between about the tenth and the seventeenth centuries CE, such advanced energy-focused practices were commonplace within Hatha Yoga sects. They found their way into the four main Hatha Yoga texts (as well as many others), the *Hatha Yoga Pradīpikā*, the *Gheranda-Samhitā*, the *Goraksha-Samhitā*, and the *Shiva-Samhitā*. Likewise, nearly every modern scholar of Yoga[15] mentions the arousal of the dormant kundalinī energy as a central goal of Hatha Yoga. I personally think an understanding of this energy, even in a theoretical sense, helps the student of Hatha Yoga see the logic behind the more common practices.

We have been exploring Hatha Yoga theory in a general sense, to help you understand the role of cleansing, strengthening muscles, developing breath control, concentrating, and relaxing in Hatha Yoga. These processes all impart benefits that amply reward the practitioner of Hatha Yoga, as attested to by the students' quotes above. Yet, in traditional Hatha Yoga these processes also prepare one for another, more advanced journey.

The Serpent Power: *Kundalinī*

I stated earlier that Hatha Yoga practice induces peak experiences in a person who has undergone adequate preparation: nonordinary, expanded, or supra-sensory states of awareness. One way that Yoga practice does this is by awakening a usually dormant (and therefore unavailable to most people)[16] energy that resides at the base of the spine. This energy is called kundalinī shakti (pronounced koon-duh-lin-ee shuk-tih), which means "coiled up energy" and is often referred to as simply kundalinī. It is represented as a snake in sacred imagery [3.5, 3.6].[17]

When this energy is aroused it often feels like pulses of heat or electricity rising in one's spine or in one's pelvis. It also creates a spectrum of experiences that vary widely from person to person. It can sometimes be disruptive, so must be approached carefully and only under expert guidance. Kundalinī arousal usually causes one's body to move involuntarily in jerks, rocking motions, gentle shaking, or by inducing head or arm movements. This experience is almost always physically pleasurable, although it can be frightening for someone who doesn't know what's happening to them. Once aroused, kundalinī shakti simply adds more energy to the vital forces one uses for living, thinking, and acting. In other words, it increases one's vitality. This increase in vitality is most useful for achieving results with the advanced concentration practices of Hatha Yoga.

Chakras, Wheels of Energy, and *Kundalinī's* Ascent

Hatha Yoga's higher concentration practices direct first the life force (prāna) and then the kundalinī

---

[15] See bibliography. One exception is T.K.V Desikachar, son of the great T Krishnamacharya. See his discussion of an alternative theory of kundalinī in *The Heart of Yoga: Developing a Personal Practice,* 138.

[16] Some Yoga authorities describe kundalinī much more generally, characterizing it as the "creative potential in man." See White (ed.), *Kundalinī, Evolution and Enlightenment,* 21–26; and Krishna, *Living with Kundalinī,* 154–155.

[17] Snakes *(nāga)* appearing in Indian art can mean many things in addition to kundalinī shakti, including deities, kings, and characters from mythology. See Crim (ed.), *The Perennial Dictionary of World Religions,* 519–520.

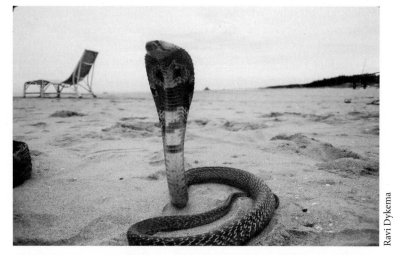

PHOTO 3.5   The aroused kundalinī energy is traditionally depicted in Indian art and sculpture as a cobra with its hood displayed.

Ravi Dykema

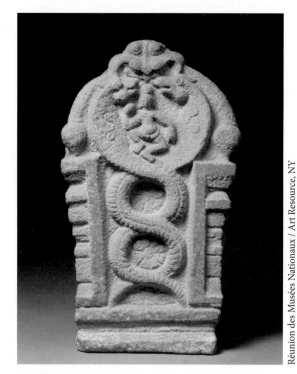

PHOTO 3.6   A stone relief sculpture of the stone serpent, Nagakal, 18th century CE.

Réunion des Musées Nationaux / Art Resource, NY

each chakra, or center, as the energy passes through it, activating the chakra's physical, emotional, mental, and psychic potential. When the kundalinī shakti passes through and opens the sixth chakra in the middle of the head, the seventh chakra at the top of the head opens automatically and one experiences samādhi, the state of unblemished pure awareness, freedom from misconception, and ecstasy.

Special Exercises to Move and Enhance Subtle Body Energy

I have been referring to many practices with which you have become familiar (and some of which I present in the next chapters) such as breathing, poses, and relaxation. In addition to these, Hatha Yoga teaches some exercises that transcend these categories and that have important uses in the management of body energy. These exercises are *mudrās* (pronounced mood-rah; seal or gesture), *kriyās* (pronounced kree-yah; actions) and *bandhas* (pronounced bahn-dha; lock). A few of them can be found in modern exercise-oriented Yoga, such as the root lock (*mūla-bandha*, pronounced moo-la bahn-dha) which involves contracting the anal sphincter muscles. Another is the horse gesture (*ashvini-mudrā*, pronounced ahsh-win-ee mood-rah), which involves repeated contraction and release of the same muscles (see Box 3.7).

You could think of these three types of Yoga exercises—mudrās, kriyās, and bandhas—as extra dials and switches on your body's control panel. These dials increase your abilities in two ways: they give you more control over *how much* energy is flowing in your body, and they give you more capacity to control the *direction* of your energy flow.

shakti into the central channel (nadī) of the spine, called *sushumnā nādī* (pronounced soo-shoom-nah nah-dee, most gracious channel). These energies, prāna and kundalinī, are directed by concentration practices to rise through the seven subtle body centers called chakras, beginning at the base of the spine and extending to the top of the head. Ideally the passage of super-charged energy opens

BOX **3.5**

The Seven Chakras, Centers of Energy

These energy centers are located in the most subtle of your five bodies (see the section "The Energy Body and the Five Bodies" earlier in this chapter), your ānanda-maya-kosha or body of bliss. The centers affect all the other bodies, too. They are essential to your personality, your emotions, your physical state, and your spiritual state.

Chakra number	Name in English and Sanskrit	Level in the body (all surrounding the spine)	Associated element	Associated feelings
1	The "root support" center, *mūlādhāra chakra* (pronounced moo-lah-dha-ra)	Base of the spine	Earth	Survival and instincts
2	The "own base" center, *svādhishthāna chakra* (pronounced swah'-dhisht-hah'-na).	Pelvis near the genitals	Water	Sexuality
3	The "jeweled city" center, *manipūra chakra* (pronounced mah-ni-poo'-ra).	Behind a spot a few inches above the navel	Fire	Power and will
4	The "un-struck sound" center, *ānāhata chakra* (pronounced ah'-nah'-ha-ta).	Near the heart	Air	Yearning and love
5	The "purity" center, *vishuddha chakra* (pronounced vi-shoo-dha).	Mid-throat	Space	Expression
6	The "command" center, *ājnā chakra* (pronounced ahj-nah).	Middle of head at level of eyebrows	Mind	Cognition and intuition
7	The "thousand-petaled lotus" center, *sahasrāra chakra* (pronounced sa-has-rah'-ra).	Top of head	No element	Feeling connected to reality, at home wherever you are

Summary of Kundalinī's Journey

You have learned the theories related to kundalinī and chakras within traditional Hatha Yoga. In brief, they are to gain control of and increase *prāna*, your life force; awaken *kundalinī*, the powerful energy, from her abode at the base of your spine; and, with it, open all of your *chakras*, or energy centers. The yogin who can do this can reliably attain *samādhi*, ecstasy, on numerous occasions. Eventually, Hatha Yoga teaches, your repeated but temporary "realizations" change your understanding of who you are and you identify more and more with your True Self, *parama-ātman*,

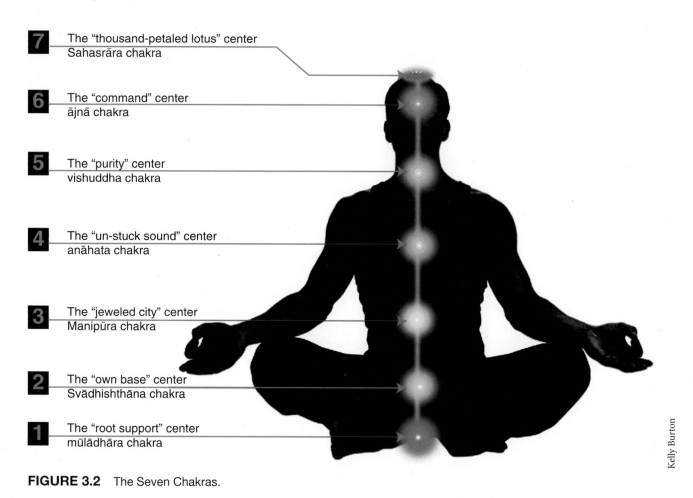

7 The "thousand-petaled lotus" center
   Sahasrāra chakra

6 The "command" center
   ājnā chakra

5 The "purity" center
   vishuddha chakra

4 The "un-stuck sound" center
   anāhata chakra

3 The "jeweled city" center
   Manipūra chakra

2 The "own base" center
   Svādhishthāna chakra

1 The "root support" center
   mūlādhāra chakra

Kelly Burton

FIGURE 3.2   The Seven Chakras.

BOX **3.6**

A Chakra Awareness Exercise

Sit cross-legged on a cushion with your back straight, or sit on a chair with your back unsupported. Bring your awareness into your body by focusing on your sensations of breathing: in your nostrils, in your throat, in your chest, and in your abdomen. After a few minutes, concentrate all your attention on your abdomen just below the base of your rib cage, about eight inches in. This is the vicinity of your third chakra, manipūra chakra. Don't worry about whether you are focusing in just the right spot. Keep holding your attention in this region, and visualize a fire burning in the place where you are focusing, like a small campfire. Maintain this visualization for five to ten minutes.

To end, become aware of your legs and arms, and notice the sounds around you.

Take some deep breaths and stretch. After a minute or so, open your eyes.

Now take an inventory of how you feel. The third chakra is related to power, will, and strength. This practice may increase your feeling of confidence that you can handle your current challenges in life. Or it may make you aware of a feeling of not having enough power, will, or strength. Either kind of awareness is useful. Just let the feelings be present in you. These effects are likely to be quite subtle, if they happen at all for you, so pay close attention to how you feel before, during, and after the exercise. It also helps to do the chakra awareness exercise every day for a week, and then write about how it affects you.

BOX **3.7**

A Mudrā Exercise: Ashwini Mudrā (Horse Gesture)

Sit in a chair or cross-legged on the floor with your back straight. Relax your weight into the floor and sense your body. Let your breath be easy and natural throughout this exercise. Now tighten your anal sphincter muscles for a moment. Then relax them. These are the muscles you use to stop the flow of urine or to stop defecation. (If you can't find them, next time you urinate, try stopping the flow, and feel which muscles you use. Most people find it easy to locate these muscles, called the pubococcygeus muscles or "floor of the pelvis muscles.") Repeat this tensing and relaxing of your pelvic floor muscles once every two seconds or so, doing fifteen repetitions total. Do this practice every day for a month, adding two repetitions each day until you are doing seventy-five repetitions. This exercise imparts many benefits to the genitals and to the pelvic floor, including increasing sensation in this region, improving blood supply, increasing muscle tone in the pelvic floor, increasing ejaculatory control, increasing energy flow in the spine and brighter awareness.

and less with your usual ego-bound self, *jīva-ātman*. In Hatha Yoga, as in Bhakti Yoga, Karma Yoga, Rāja Yoga or any of the other Yoga schools, the goal is the same: true knowing, seeing reality (and yourself) as it truly is. And all of the practices in the system move step by step toward that goal.

Applying Hatha Yoga Theory in Your Yoga practice

I said at the beginning of this chapter that through studying traditional Hatha Yoga theory, we can understand how modern "daughter" Yoga systems draw from, and expand on the traditional system. Modern Yoga systems usually contain four essential components of traditional Hatha Yoga practice: poses that you move through or hold, breath awareness, relaxation practices, and meditation. (We explore these in the next three chapters.) And modern Yoga usually incorporates key elements of Hatha Yoga theory: clarity, control and surrender (see pages 39–42).

Here's how this works: when you perform Yoga poses and Yoga breathing you feel your muscles working. You feel your breath flowing in and out, getting deeper. You feel the sensation of stretching your spine and joints, increasing your blood circulation and respiration (clarity, p. 39). As you continue practicing and feeling all these sensations (control, p. 40) your mind becomes quieter. The quieter your mind gets, the more you feel/experience yourself in the moment. Then your intimate moment-to-moment experience guides your movement and breath. It guides your level of effort or of relaxation. This dialogue between your practice and your body's feedback leads to, in many cases, a deeper and deeper and progressively clearer connection with your whole self: your felt experience, your flow of thoughts, your emotions and moods. For most people this is hugely rejuvenating and joyous (surrender, p. 42). This connection to your whole self can last for hours, days, or even weeks after an especially potent Yoga practice session. This is the state of "balanced energy," that the name, "Hatha Yoga" alludes to.

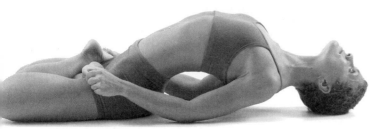

Goodman Photography

Yoga Breathing

Introduction to Yoga Breathing (*Prānāyāma*)

Hatha Yoga and its offshoot, modern exercise-oriented Yoga, are both best known for their postures that stretch, strengthen, and relax your body. Yet the scholarly and scriptural literature of Hatha Yoga suggest that breath practices are just as important as postures, if not more so. As you read on the next page (Box 4.1), the old yogic teaching emphasizes breath control practices, prānāyāma, as the central way for a yogin to purify his physical and energy body, to build strength and stamina, to control his mind, and to achieve clear perception. We can view many other types of Hatha Yoga practice, such as Yoga poses, as training for breath control—as a conditioning program so that the yogin's breath control techniques will work as they are designed to.[1]

A Hatha yogin's first breath-related goal is to slow down his breath and to make his inhalations and exhalations even. His next goal is to learn to hold his breath briefly during each breath cycle. Stopping his breath is the way he stops his constant mental turmoil. His mental turmoil obscures his view of reality, making his view of things foggy and even distorted.

The yogin's second breath-related goal is to use his newfound strength, stamina, and breathing skill to alter his awareness, and achieve super-happy or super-clear states of mind.

The kind of yogin I am describing is rare today. Not many Yoga students undertake extensive training in a traditional Hatha Yoga school. Most people taking a yoga class will never need to know how to stop their breath for 32 seconds (a traditional benchmark), or how to slow their breath down to the rate of one breath per minute, and sustain that for two hours.[2] Yoga students today who are seeking better health, increased powers of concentration, and more energy can still benefit from the sophisticated understanding of breathing contained in the Hatha Yoga system. Yoga contains many simple, safe, and easy breath practices that have useful effects on anyone who

---

[1] Prānāyāma is also much older than poses (āsanas), which date from the Tantric era. The first written record of prānāyāma practices is in the *Atharva-Veda,* fifteenth book (2000 BCE), which mentions the "apparent practice of prānāyāma and other similar austerities." Feuerstein, *The Yoga Tradition* , 121.

---

[2] For more descriptions ot traditional breathing training see Bernard, *Hatha Yoga,* 54–70.

> **BOX 4.1**
>
> # Scholars and Sages on Breath Control (*Prānāyāma*)
>
> There is no austerity which leads higher than breath control. It purifies all impurity and the flame of knowledge is kindled.
>
> —Vyasa, in *Yoga-Bhashya*
> (a fifth-century commentary on the *Yoga Sūtra*)[3]
>
> There is always a connection between respiration and mental states.
>
> —King Bhoja, in *Raja-martananda*
> (an eleventh-century commentary
> on the *Yoga Sūtra*)[4]
>
> Yogins hold that prāna [vital energy] is the force behind the renewal of the body cells, and that disease is unlikely to gain a hold on a body whose every cell is permeated with pranic [vital] energy. Further, a body freshly charged with prāna can be a source of healing for others, by transmission.
>
> —James Hewitt, in *The Complete Yoga Book*[5]
>
> Prānāyāma [breath control] reinforces the power of meditative practices, and it is upon this technique that the Tantras [ancient texts of Tantra Yoga] lay the strongest emphasis.
>
> —Ajit Mookerjee, in *Kundalinī,
> the Arousal of the Inner Energy*[6]

practices them. I will cover a number of them here.

As with all Yoga practices, I recommend learning from a living teacher. This is especially important in the case of Yoga breathing.

Yoga Breath Practices (*Yoga Prānāyāmas*)

Practice Guidelines

Yoga breathing is safe and effective when it is done properly. The key to safe practice is to avoid straining. When you are breathing on purpose you should feel comfortable; the effort required should feel slight. Since normal breathing is automatic and therefore effortless, breathing on purpose (called voluntary breathing) will feel weird to some people. It takes a little while to get used to. If you feel the need to get more air, such as to breathe faster, or if you feel agitated, tense, dizzy, or uncomfortable, you should abandon the control for the moment and let your breath be automatic. When, after a minute or two, your breathing feels normal and comfortable again, you may start the breath control once more. Don't attempt it a third time. Do try it again the next day. The same practice may feel fine by then. If it doesn't, consult your teacher.

One way that I guide students to take it easy with breath is to recommend that they get a *C* for effort. This requires that, for most of us, we'll have to feel like lazy Yoga students.

[3] Danielou, Yoga: Mastering the Secrets of Matter and the Universe, 82.

[4] Eliade, Patanjali and Yoga, 69.

[5] Hewitt, *The Complete Yoga Book,* 123.

[6] Mookerjee, *Kundalini: the Arousal of the Inner Energy,* 19.

BOX **4.2**

Students' Comments on the Effects of Yoga Breathing

These quotes are from papers written by Yoga students at Naropa University.

A woman student from Latvia writes: "[Yoga breathing] is very beneficial for me because I tend to 'overreact,' especially while speaking in public, reading my poems to an audience, etc. I develop an unpleasant 'neurotic fever': trembling hands and legs, uncontrollable voice. Now I have started to use lower-lung breath [taught below] and it helps! I am getting more self-confident and able to reduce my negative physical reaction."

A male graduate student writes: "Something profound has happened to me since I began inhaling, holding the in-breath for six counts, then exhaling and holding the out-breath for six counts. When I fill my lungs with air and hold I feel elated, as if I am about to leap. I am suspended above a realm of possibilities. It's a comfortable feeling. Then comes time to let go, to let the air out of my lungs and hold. The first time I did this particular practice, I panicked. I wanted to pull air into my lungs as quickly as possible, whether I needed it or not. The discomfort had very little to do with lack of oxygen. To breathe out is to relax. I was having a hard time relaxing. I always have a hard time relaxing. Why? . . . The more I held the breath out—and tried to relax—the more I came to feel this incredible sense of loss for so many things. The loss I felt seemed deeper than my own personal history. The anguish and sorrow over the death of my marriage came to me not as my own personal loss, but as if I was mourning the extinction of a rare species—the knowledge that something had been lost in this universe, something that will never be again. This feeling rippled out to everything else; from the death of my grandmothers to the yellowing pages for a book of poetry on my bookshelf. . . . What's left? Breathe it out. Relax."

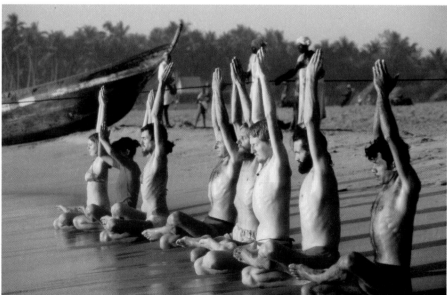

© Ravi Dykema

PHOTO 4.1   Students performing Yoga breath practices on a beach in India.

> ## BOX 4.3
>
> # Checklist of Yoga Breath Guidelines
>
> - Don't strain.
> - Get a *C* for effort; be lazy, but perform the exercise precisely.
> - Stop if you feel dizzy or uncomfortable. Try again later or the next day.
> - Don't compete with other students.
> - Keep some of your attention on relaxing, especially the muscles that you aren't using for breathing.
> - Don't hold your breath for more than a brief pause until you are experienced with Yoga breathing.
> - Do only those practices that are for your level of expertise.

If you catch yourself putting out 100 percent, "going for it," or competing with another student, back off. Continue to perform the practice with precision, using the effort needed to follow the directions. Yet always keep some of your attention on relaxing, even while the bulk of your focus is on doing. Especially relax the muscles that aren't involved in the exercise, like your face, your lower jaw, your arms, your shoulders, and your legs. This is also the formula for allowing energy to flow (see "'Letting Go' in the Practice of Yoga Poses and Yoga Breathing," Chapter 3).

Don't attempt prānāyāmas that are beyond your level. Start with beginning practices and progress step by step. A good general rule is to only do practices that incorporate in and out breathing, with no breath holding, or at least only very short pauses after the in or out breath. Only do prānāyāmas that involve breath holding if you learn them from an experienced teacher.

Basic Proper Breathing

Automatic and Voluntary Breathing

Your body breathes for you. You don't need to think about inhaling or do anything about it. You don't even need to know that you are breathing.

You breathe when you are asleep or unconscious. Breathing is automatic; like your heart beating or your skin sweating, it is part of the functioning of your *autonomic nervous system,* which is controlled by your brain. But unlike your heartbeat and your sweat, you can, if you choose, take control of your breathing, making it voluntary. When you do this in the proper fashion you benefit your nervous system, your circulatory system, your lymph system, and your muscular system. These benefits occur because of the increase in oxygen (and decrease in carbon dioxide) in your bloodstream. These benefits also result from the muscular action of breathing and the relaxation induced by slow breathing.

Many of these changes are incidental to the purposes for which breath was used in Hatha Yoga, that is, expanding awareness, but they are useful to the person living an ordinary life in the world.

Yoga breathing, and any other kind of voluntary breathing, should be done only occasionally and only for short periods. Your body *needs* autonomic breath to regulate itself. A beginner to Yoga breathing should practice controlling her breath no more than fifteen minutes per day, building up to thirty minutes by the end of two months of regular practice. An experienced yogin may spend a few hours per day doing Yoga prānāyāma, but the rest of the day she lets her breath operate autonomi-cally. She *may pay attention to* her breathing many more hours per day, sensing her breathing (a Yoga mindfulness practice), but she doesn't try to change it. She lets it be automatic.

Natural Breath Awareness: The Autonomic Breath

Preparation   The corpse pose or the modified corpse pose (*shava-āsana,* pronounced shav ah-sa-na) [4.2 and 4.3]. Lie on a firm, yet comfortable surface, such as a thick blanket folded in half lengthwise or several sticky mats. Lie with your knees bent or with your legs straight, whichever you like better. If bent, your knees and feet should be slightly apart, about the same as the width of your hips. If straight, your legs should be comfortably close together. Rest your arms on the floor at your sides, or bend your elbows a little and rest your hands on your hips or upper thighs. Close your eyes.

The Exercise   Bring your attention gently to your sensations of heaviness. Feel the points where your body presses into the floor, and surrender to the floor. Let the floor support your head, your back, your buttocks, your legs, and your arms.

After a few minutes of this focus, shift your attention to your breathing sensations. Feel your belly moving,

your chest moving, and your back moving in rhythm with your breath. Breathing is the most obvious sign that you are alive. It started when you emerged from your mother's womb and won't stop till you "breathe your last."

Continue this focus for a while. Continue exploring the sensations made by your moving breath, such as the rush of air past your nostrils, into your throat, and down into your chest. Notice that it is cool when rushing in, and warm when flowing out. You may feel the swelling of your belly as you inhale at one moment, and the air-flow in your throat the next. Notice the sensations in the muscles you use to breathe: muscles in the base of your ribs, in your mid-chest, in your back, and in your shoulders and neck (see Figures 4.1 and 4.2). Feel your muscles with both your inhalation and your exhalation.

It is OK to tour your body, or to stay with one sensation for a while. Just keep your attention on *some* sensation of breathing. If your mind wanders, that's OK. When you notice that your attention is somewhere other than on breath, just bring it back to your breath. This may happen over and over. That's OK. Just keep coming back to your breath.

To Finish   After five to ten minutes, take some purposeful deep breaths, stretch your arms and legs, and then roll onto your side. After a few seconds, slowly sit up.

Benefits   Sensing your breath quiets your mind. Notice that when you are really engrossed in a breath sensation, your usual mental chatter is silent. This may happen only for an instant, whereupon the thoughts return. But it usually does happen. See if you can spot it. Relief from mental chatter is soothing and calming.

You may not be able to hear your mental chatter, your flow of thoughts, yet. You may notice,

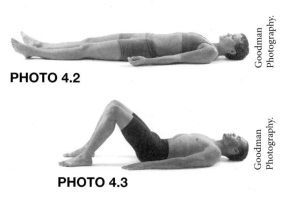

PHOTO 4.2

Goodman Photography.

PHOTO 4.3

Goodman Photography.

Muscles of respiration

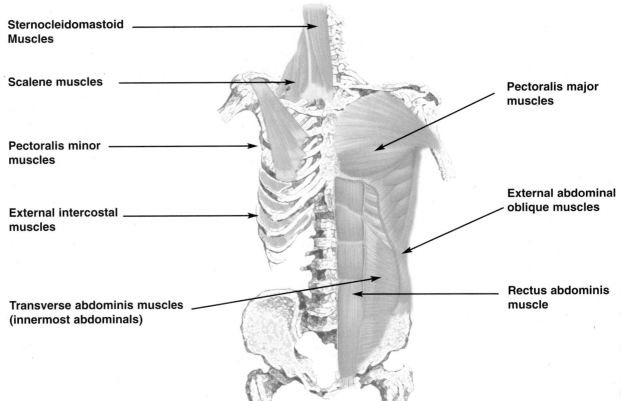

Sternocleidomastoid Muscles

Scalene muscles

Pectoralis minor muscles

External intercostal muscles

Transverse abdominis muscles (innermost abdominals)

Pectoralis major muscles

External abdominal oblique muscles

Rectus abdominis muscle

Kelly Burton/Cengage Learning

FIGURE 4.1   The physiology of breathing in and out.
The muscles that create deep inhalations: Your diaphragm draws your lungs downward, filling the lower part of your lungs; the muscles between your ribs (external intercostal muscles) expand your chest's circumference, drawing air into your lower, middle, and upper lungs; and the muscles in your upper chest and neck (sternocleidomastoid, scalene, and pectoralis minor muscles) pull your upper ribs and collarbone upward. For exhalation muscles, see the caption under Figure 4.2.

though, that you become calmer as you observe your breath sensations, and that your breathing slows down. This slowing of your breath rate relaxes and calms you.

Your automatic breath is your friend and comforter. Get to know her. Invite her in for tea. Listen to her stories. She may seem boring at first, but I predict that soon she'll seem wise and loving.

Diaphragmatic Breath #1, Adham Prānāyāma

Also called "lower lung breath," this is the first part of a four-part practice called *Vibhaga Prānāyāma* (pronounced vib-ha-ga prah-nah-yah-ma), which literally means "chapter breathing" or "sectional

breathing." It includes, in addition to diaphragmatic breathing, intercostal breathing, clavicular breathing, and complete breathing.

Prerequisite   Only begin this practice, which involves voluntary breathing, after you have spent some time over a number of days with the autonomic breath, taught previously.

Preparation   Assume the modified corpse pose, shava-āsana [4.3]: Place a mat or blanket on the floor, as above. Lie on your back with your knees bent ninety degrees and slightly apart, about the same width as your hips. Your bare feet rest on the mat, also hip-width apart. Place your hands over your lower rib cage, so

The diaphragm movement in breathing

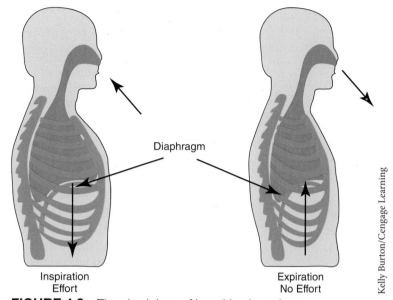

Diaphragm

Inspiration
Effort

Expiration
No Effort

Kelly Burton/Cengage Learning

FIGURE 4.2   The physiology of breathing in and out.
The muscles that create rapid exhalations (normal exhalations require no muscle effort at all) are (in Figure 4.1) the abdominal muscles (external abdominal oblique, rectus abdominis, internal abdominal oblique [not shown], and transverse abdominis). These muscles compress your abdomen to squeeze up from underneath your lungs, exhaling air from your lower lungs. The muscles between your ribs (internal intercostal muscles, beneath the ones shown) shrink your chest's circumference, squeezing air out of your lower, middle, and upper lungs.

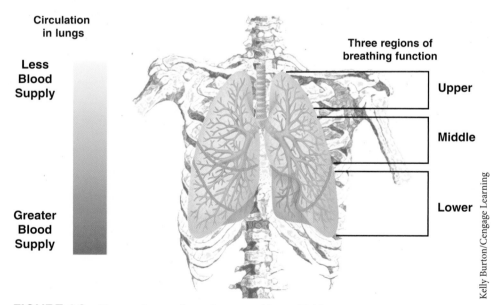

Circulation in lungs

Less Blood Supply

Greater Blood Supply

Three regions of breathing function

Upper

Middle

Lower

Kelly Burton/Cengage Learning

FIGURE 4.3   The anatomy of your lungs and bronchial tree.
Your lungs consist of three lobes on the right and two on the left. Your breathing function, however, is divided into three zones on both sides equally—lower, middle, and upper. Note the greater blood supply to the lower lungs, thus the importance of diaphragmatic (lower) breathing for more efficient gaseous exchange between your blood and the air you've inhaled (carbon dioxide exchanged for oxygen).[7]

[7] Coulter, *Anatomy of Hatha Yoga*, 106.

your little fingers are just below your lowest ribs. Rest your elbows on the floor. Close your eyes [4.4].

The Exercise   Relax your weight into the floor, sensing the places where you feel pressure against the floor. This releases your most easily accessed tensions. Stay with this for a few minutes.

Shift your attention to your breath sensations. Put your main focus under your hands in your lower chest. Now intentionally send your breath under your hands, so that your belly puffs up toward the ceiling when you *inhale,* and drops down toward the floor when you *exhale.* You can feel the movement of your belly with your little fingers, and in your belly itself [4.5 and 4.6].

If this doesn't happen, or if this movement is slight, notice your upper and middle chest, which will likely be

moving noticeably with each breath. See if you can keep your upper chest still, while you use *only* your lower chest and your belly to draw in the breath. Drop your belly toward the floor as you *exhale.* Then as soon as you start the next *in breath,* release your belly and let it puff up toward the ceiling. Although you don't actually breathe in your abdomen, your abdomen's movements are a key to releasing your diaphragm.

Continue breathing in your lower lungs (or attempting to) in this fashion for five to ten minutes, focusing under your hands and feeling your breathing sensations. When your mind wanders to a thought and you are no longer focusing on the exercise, just bring your focus back to what you are doing. This may happen over and over. That's OK.

This gets easier and easier with practice, and your sensations will become more vivid and detailed. As they become more vivid and interesting your attention will wander less.

To Finish   End your control of your breath and return to autonomic, effortless breathing, noticing how this transition feels. After a minute, stretch as you take some deep breaths, then roll on your side to sit up.

Benefits   See below, after "Diaphragmatic Breath #3," for benefits.

Diaphragmatic Breath #2, the Pelvic Tilt

Preparation   The modified corpse pose, shava-āsana [4.3], the same as for Breath #1.

The Exercise   After doing Diaphragmatic Breath #1 for a few minutes, add a spinal movement and pelvic tilt in sync with your breath. Here's how: As you start to *exhale,* rock your pelvis so that the waistline part of your back drops toward the floor. Your lower back may even touch the

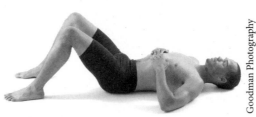

PHOTO 4.4

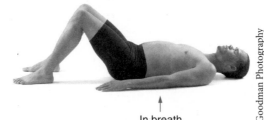

In breath
PHOTO 4.5   Note the movement of the belly as you inhale and exhale.

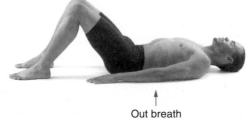

Out breath
PHOTO 4.6

Goodman Photography

floor as you complete your exhalation [4.7]. As you *inhale,* let your pelvis

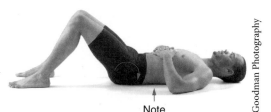

Note

PHOTO 4.7 Exhaling, rock your pelvis so that your lower back drops toward the floor.

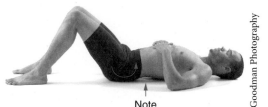

Note

PHOTO 4.8 Inhaling, let your pelvis rock back to where it came from.

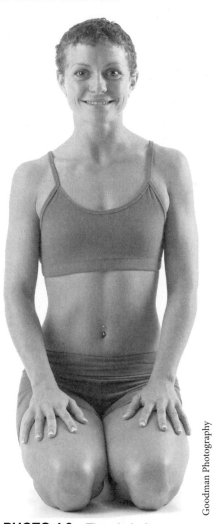

PHOTO 4.9 Thunderbolt pose, vajra āsana.

rock back to where it came from, and your lower back will arch slightly upwards, to its prior position [4.8].

Don't press into the floor with your feet in order to rock your pelvis. Let your legs rest, your feet relaxing into the floor. The muscle action that creates this movement is only in your abdomen. Your back, buttocks, and legs stay relaxed.

Continue this breath/movement, tipping your pelvis as you *exhale* so your lower back descends toward and even presses the floor, and releasing this effort as you *inhale* so your pelvis untilts; that is, it returns to its "neutral" position, as does your back. Please continue focusing under your hands into your lower lungs, feeling your belly puff out (up toward the ceiling) with each *inhalation,* and drop toward the floor with each *exhalation.* Continue for five to ten minutes. When your mind wanders to a thought and you are no longer focusing on the exercise, just bring your focus back to what you are doing. This may happen over and over. That's OK.

To Finish End your control of your breath and return to autonomic, effortless breathing, noticing how this transition feels. After a minute, stretch as you take some deep breaths, then roll onto your side to sit up.

Benefits See below, after "Diaphragmatic Breath #3," for benefits.

Diaphragmatic Breath #3, the Sitting Lower Lung Breath

Preparation The thunderbolt pose (*vajra āsana,* pronounced vah-jrah ah-sa-na) [4.9].

Fold a blanket in fourths to create a sitting pad, or use a couple of folded towels. Kneel on the pad with your feet and knees together. Lower your buttocks toward your heels, letting your heels separate slightly, about eight inches apart. Sit on your heels, resting

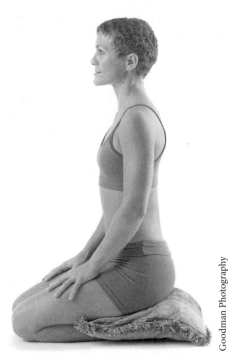

PHOTO 4.10

Goodman Photography

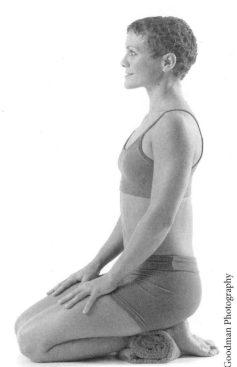

PHOTO 4.11

Goodman Photography

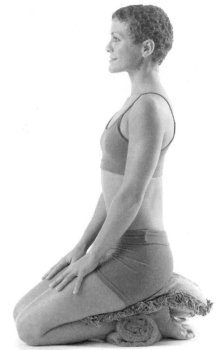

PHOTO 4.12

Goodman Photography

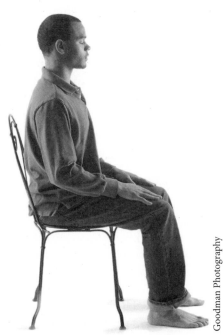

PHOTO 4.13   An alternative to the thunderbolt pose, for Yoga breathing.

Goodman Photography

you weight into your legs and feet. Sit erect so your back is in a position such as when you are standing. Adjust your buttocks' position on your heels so you can achieve this erect posture.

Pointers   If your knees hurt right away, or after a short while in the position, adjust the pose by placing a pillow, folded blanket, or rolled up towel on top of your calves and feet, between your buttocks and feet [4.10]. This reduces the bend in your knees. If your ankles hurt, place a rolled up towel or small pillow under your ankles [4.11]. Or support both your ankles and knees [4.12].

When to Do an Alternate Pose   If none of these adjustments makes the thunderbolt pose comfortable or at least tolerable, assume an alternate pose. Sit on a chair, your feet flat on the floor hip-width apart, with your back erect, not leaning back in the chair [4.13].

More Preparation   Sit in this position for a minute or two, with your hands resting palms-down on your thighs, and sense you body. Relax your weight downward, feeling any sensations that appear to you.

Further prepare for Yoga breathing by sensing and relaxing areas of tension that interfere with diaphragmatic breathing: Notice your lower jaw; relax it. Let your tongue relax. Your mouth may open slightly. Notice your throat; relax it. Notice your belly; relax it. Let it swell with your inhalations. Notice the floor of your pelvis (your anal sphincter muscles); relax it. Notice your legs; relax them.

The Exercise   Place your hands on your lower rib cage, so your little fingers are just below your lowest ribs, your thumbs under your breasts [4.14]. Relax your shoulders. Position your head on top of your neck as if you were looking straight ahead. Close your eyes.

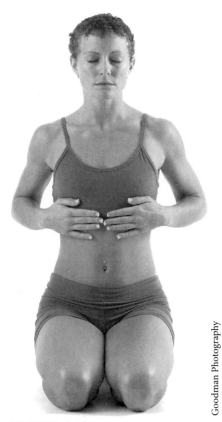

PHOTO 4.14

Goodman Photography

Bring your attention to your hands, then under your hands, through your ribs, into your chest. Let your breath drop into the bottom of your lungs, as you did in Exercise #2, so that your belly expands as you *inhale,* and draws in as you *exhale.* Breathe a little more deeply than you would if you breathed automatically. Notice that as you *inhale* your chest expands under your hands. Let your upper chest be still. Concentrate your breath, as best you can, in just your lower chest and belly. As you breathe, sense the sides and back of your lower rib cage too, and let them expand and shrink with each breath.

Continue this exercise for three minutes, about fifteen breaths.

To Finish   Rest you hands on your thighs again, and let your breathing return to automatic. You may naturally sigh, yawn, or take a deep breath, or even breathe shallowly. Let any of these things happen. Feel your sensations as your breath becomes automatic.

Benefits of Diaphragmatic Breath (Numbers 1, 2, and 3)

Effects on Your Abdominal Organs
The lower lung breath is accomplished by contractions in your diaphragm and intercostal (between the ribs) muscles (Figures 4.1–4.3). The most important of these two muscle groups, as far as the effects of this breath are concerned, is the diaphragm.

Each time your diaphragm *contracts* to create an inhalation, it presses down on the abdominal cavity and its contents—your liver, kidneys, spleen, stomach, intestines, and so on. When you exhale, your diaphragm *relaxes* and rises upward, drawn up by the elasticity of the lungs, releasing the pressure on your abdominal cavity. This cycle of pressure-release massages your abdominal organs, increasing blood circulation and

improving digestion/elimination. This press-release cycle also reveals to you when you are holding unconscious tension. For example you may be unconsciously holding in your abdomen. If you become aware of this you may be able to release it. The next time you have a stomachache, try the diaphragmatic breathing exercises and see what happens. Some people have reported that their stomach ache goes away.

Effects on Your Energy and Awareness
The lower lung breath energizes your lower belly, your pelvis, and your arms and legs. Lower breath makes it easier to feel these areas. It helps you feel emotions that inhabit your belly and pelvis, such as anger, hatred, wanting, willfulness, and sexual desire (these are often called visceral emotions). This breath helps you access your creativity—your desire to do or to create.

Effects on Your Nervous System
Diaphragmatic breath (lower lung breath) engages the parasympathetic nervous system, whereas mid- and upper-chest breath engages your sympathetic nervous system. This means that lower lung breath relaxes you, lowers your blood pressure, increases digestion, awakens your internal sensations, makes you aware of your emotions, and enables your mind to think of many possibilities. All these effects accompany the functioning of your parasympathetic nervous system, which you use when you are feeling safe and comfortable.

Your "emergency" nervous system, which kicks in when your life is in danger (or when you think it is), is called your sympathetic nervous system. This nervous system takes over your whole body and makes you feel different and function differently from when you are using your parasympathetic system. This system can be partially engaged (as when

BOX 4.4

The Two Nervous Systems

Sympathetic Nervous System	Parasympathetic Nervous System
Rapid mid and upper lung breathing	Slower diaphragmatic breath
Anxious and agitated	Unafraid, relaxed, and comfortable
Numb to inner emotion and sensations	Aware of inner sensations and emotion
External awareness amplified	Outer and inner awareness *both* available
Thoughts revolve around finding the danger, now	Thoughts free to consider anything, now or later
Ability to consider few options: all options relate to "freeze, fight, or flee"	Ability to consider many options
Feeling "I'll be overwhelmed"	Feeling "I can handle it"
Digestion inhibited	Digestion functioning normally
Blood pressure rises	Blood pressure normal
Heart rate increases	Heart rate normal

you breathe in your mid and upper lungs), creating subtle effects, or fully engaged, creating dramatic effects. The dramatic effects of sympathetic nervous system function are sweaty hands and feet (to run and climb with), rapid intercostal breathing (mid and upper), inhibited digestion, reduction of internal sensation and emotion, acute external awareness (especially sight and hearing), mental anticipation of threat (your mind searches for or focuses on the source of the threat), and access to limited options—freeze, fight, or flee.

If you hear a scary noise in the bushes at night, you flip into your sympathetic nervous system. Your splitting headache goes away completely. Your sadness because your boyfriend/girlfriend just left you disappears. You can hear every sound and see much better in the dark. You can't think about the future, only the now. And you are frozen with fear, ready to instantly fight or run. Your bloodstream is loaded with adrenaline. Your body can handle this fine if it happens only occasionally. But many of us live with our sympathetic nervous systems partly engaged most

of the time. This predisposes us to heart attacks, stomach problems, high blood pressure, and other health problems.[8] Diaphragmatic breathing can be helpful to us.

Here's a practical example. When your mother gets unjustly mad at you, you start out being silent and motionless, feeling nothing, staring into space (freeze). Then eventually you end up yelling angrily (fight) and slamming the door as you leave (flight). You're in your sympathetic nervous system. Your nervous system gives you only those three options. They may help you when a bear is attacking you, but they aren't helpful for intimate relationships. Try going off by yourself—breathe in your lower lungs for five minutes; get into your parasympathetic nervous system. Then come back to your mother, able to feel and describe your own emotions and empathize with hers, able to consider many options (only *one of which* is to run out and slam the door). In your parasympathetic

---

[8] Coulter, *Anatomy of Hatha Yoga*, 105, 108. Also see Douillard, *Perfect Health for Kids*, 299.

system you feel safer, more comfortable, less threatened, and more able to handle whatever comes.

Remember that in Chapter 3 (under the heading "'Letting Go' in the Practice of Yoga Poses and Yoga Breathing," page 44), we explored the requirement that yogins be able to tolerate intense sensation, energy flows, and states of arousal. To do this yogins need to be able to stay in their parasympathetic nervous systems. Diaphragmatic breathing is essential for accomplishing that.

Intercostal Breath #1, Madhya Prānāyāma

Also called "middle lung breath," this is the second part of the four-part practice called Vibhaga Prānāyāma, "sectional breathing." It includes, in addition to intercostal breathing, diaphragmatic breathing, clavicular breathing, and complete breathing.

Prerequisite   The development of some skill in performing diaphragmatic breath, taught earlier.

Preparation   Lie in the modified corpse pose, shava-āsana [4.3]. Close your eyes. Sense your weight pressing into the floor. Surrender to the floor. Relax your forehead, your lower jaw, your arms, and your belly. Place your hands on your breasts, your fingers close together, with your elbows resting on the floor, your shoulders relaxed [4.15].

The Exercise   Focus into your hands. Then move your focus downward through skin, breasts, muscles, ribs, into your middle lungs. Keep you

focus there and purposely breathe, intending for the air to go under your hands, into your middle lungs. Check that you are *not* using your diaphragm, *not* puffing your belly out on your in breath. This is exclusively a middle lung breath. Keep focusing under your hands, and keep breathing voluntarily, a little more deeply than you would with automatic breath.

Continue this for about ten breaths. Then focus into the sides and back of the same region—your middle lungs. Send the air to these areas, too. When you breathe to the back it feels as if you are breathing against the floor. Continue this fuller middle breath for another ten to fifteen breaths, about five minutes. Your mind will probably wander to thoughts or to a sound you hear. That's OK. Just bring your attention gently back to your middle breath, over and over.

To Finish   Drop your hands to the floor at your sides. End the controlled breath, letting your breath become automatic. See where the air wants to go, into which parts of your lungs. Stay with this for a few moments, stretch, roll on your side, and sit up.

Benefits   The intercostal breath helps you feel the difference between middle breath, which engages muscles between your ribs, and diaphragmatic breath. It builds your skill toward being able to do a complete breath. It energizes your mid-body from your navel to your throat, especially vitalizing your lungs and heart. It helps you feel heart emotions, like empathy, love, compassion, sadness, yearning, envy, and jealousy.

Intercostal Breath #2, Madhya Prānāyāma

Preparation   Assume the thunderbolt pose, vajra āsana [4.9, or with props, 4.10–4.12] or sit in a chair [4.13].

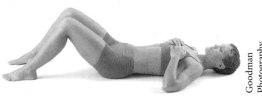

PHOTO 4.15

Goodman Photography

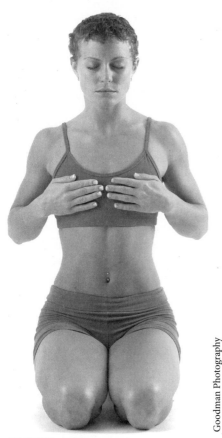

PHOTO 4.16

Goodman Photography

Relax in this pose, and sense your weight passing down through your body into the floor. Place your hands over your breasts, as you did in Intercostal Breath #1, your fingers close together, letting your elbows relax near your sides [4.16].

The Exercise   Focus into your hands, then through your chest wall into your middle lungs. Keep focusing inside your lungs, right under your hands, and intend for your breath to come here. Don't try to make it happen. Just relax, focus, and intend to breathe where you are focusing. Include your sides and back in your focus, so each breath expands your chest in all directions. The air will tend to go wherever you place your attention. Breathe a little more deeply than you would with automatic breath.

Continue this middle breath for five minutes, about fifteen breaths. Retrieve your wandering mind as you did for #1.

To Finish   Place your hands on your thighs. Stop controlling your breath, letting your breath become automatic. See where the air wants to go, into what parts of your lungs, rapidly or slowly, erratically or regularly. Stay with this for a few moments. Then stretch as you take some deep breaths. Relax off your heels into a comfortable sitting position.

Benefits   This breath imparts the same benefits as #1, only more so, because you are able to breathe more deeply sitting up than you are lying down.

Clavicular Breath #1, Adhyam Prānāyāma

Also called "upper lung breath," this is the third part of the four-part practice called Vibhaga Prānāyāma, "sectional breathing."

Prerequisite   Familiarity with diaphragmatic and intercostal breathing practices.

Preparation   Assume the modified corpse pose, shava-āsana [4.3]. Close your eyes. Relax into the floor for a minute, sensing your body. Place your hands over your upper chest, above your breasts, with your fingertips crossing your collar bone (clavicle). Rest your elbows on the floor, relaxing your arms and shoulders [4.17].

The Exercise   Focus into your hands, then beneath them through your chest wall into your upper lungs. Keep your attention there, intending to draw air into this area. Relax and let it happen; don't try. As you continue this breath, spread your attention into your armpits and into your upper back as well as under your hands. Send your upper breath in all three directions, expanding all the way around with each *in breath,* and squeezing the air from all sides of this area with the *out breath.* Be sure to empty this area thoroughly before you start the next inhalation. Your inhalation may raise your shoulders slightly, especially as you fill a little more at the end. Let this happen. These muscles pull up on your clavicle and upper ribs, to admit more air.

Continue this upper lung breath for fifteen to twenty breaths, or five minutes. Keep retrieving your wandering mind, bringing your attention back to performing this breath, and feeling it.

To Finish   Rest your arms beside you on the floor and resume automatic breathing, noticing where in your

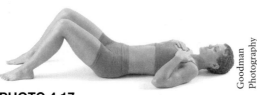

PHOTO 4.17

Goodman Photography

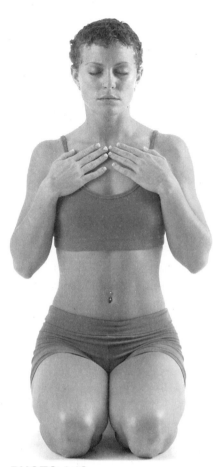

PHOTO 4.18

Goodman Photography

lungs you breathe. After a minute, stretch with a few deep breaths and roll on your side to sit up.

Benefits Emptying your upper lungs thoroughly makes it easier to breathe in all the other areas. Upper breath helps you achieve the complete breath. It clarifies the boundaries of the section below it, the middle lungs. It energizes your head, your senses, and your perception itself. Upper breath turns the lights up a little brighter. It can also enhance creativity.

Clavicular Breath #2, Adhyam Prāṇāyāma

Preparation Assume the thunderbolt pose, vajra āsana [4.9, or with props, 4.10–4.12] or sit in a chair [4.13]. Relax in this pose, and sense your weight passing down through your body into the floor, or into the chair seat. Place your hands as you did in #1, on your upper chest above your breasts, so your fingertips cross your collar bone. Your fingers will aim upward slightly when you relax your elbows downward next to your sides [4.18].

The Exercise Focus under your hands through your chest wall into your upper lungs. Feel into the sides of your upper lungs, near your armpits, and into the back of your upper lungs, near the inside of your shoulder blades, as well as in the front of your upper lungs. Send your breath where you are focusing, relaxing and letting the air move easily. Breathe a little more deeply than you would if you breathed in this area automatically. Continue this upper lung breath for five minutes, about fifteen to twenty breaths.

Pointer This is the hardest area to feel and to control for most people. Be patient. Regular practice will reward you with new sensitivity and new breathing skills.

To Finish Rest your hands on your thighs and let go of controlling your breath. Notice how and where you breathe as you resume automatic breathing. When you feel ready to, stretch to some deep sighing breaths. Then relax into a more comfortable sitting position.

Benefits This breath imparts the same benefits as Clavicular Breath #1, only more so, because you are able to breathe more deeply and with more precision sitting up than you are lying down.

Complete Breath #1, Mahat Yoga Prāṇāyāma

This breath, which literally means "great yoga breath" or "great unifying breath," is also called "three-part breathing." This is the fourth part of the four-part practice called Vibhaga Prāṇāyāma, "sectional breathing."

Prerequisite Experience with breathing into each of the three sections of your lungs, diaphragmatic, intercostal, and clavicular.

Preparation Lie in the corpse pose or the modified corpse pose [4.2 and 4.3]. Sense yourself for a few moments. Place your right hand on the center of your lower lungs and your left hand on the center of your middle lungs, between your breasts. Rest your elbows on the floor. Close your eyes [4.19].

The Exercise Inhale in three parts, as follows: First exhale completely. Then start filling under your right hand, your lower lungs; without a pause fill under your left hand, your middle lungs; then fill your upper lungs. You

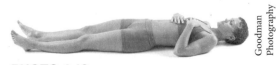

Goodman Photography

PHOTO 4.19

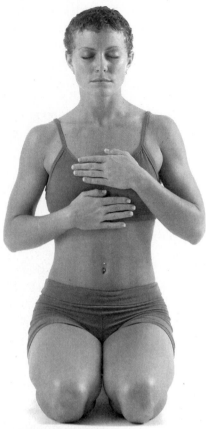

PHOTO 4.20

Goodman Photography

must *move your focus* from section to section to get the breath to move in this sequence. *Exhale* in three parts, as follows: Start emptying under your right hand, from your lower lungs; continue emptying under your left hand, from your middle lungs; then continue emptying your upper lungs, squeezing all the air out.

Continue your focus and breathe in this pattern. Remember to get a *C* for effort. Breathe lazily, yet precisely. If you start feeling short of air or tense, stop for a few breaths and then try it again.

To Finish   After twenty breaths or five to seven minutes, give up all your breathing effort. Just lie there, letting your breath do whatever it wants to. In about two minutes, stretch your arms and legs, and then roll onto your side in order to sit up.

Benefits   Complete breathing activates your parasympathetic nervous system, similarly to diaphragmatic breath (which it includes). The benefits of diaphragmatic breathing apply here, too. Complete three-part breathing ventilates your lungs and bloodstream as efficiently as it can be done, thereby increasing your blood oxygen content and decreasing your blood carbon dioxide content. This is called mild hyperventilation or over-ventilation. Deep breathing like this increases your energy and spreads it throughout your body, to your legs and arms, your pelvis and belly, your chest, your shoulders and back, and your neck and head. Every part of you is easier to feel after doing deep breathing. Complete breath clears you mind and increases your power of concentration. The practice of postures, āsanas, after deep breathing is enhanced because you can feel your muscles and joints more intimately, and you can perhaps even feel your energy flows. Any other breath

practice or posture you do is enhanced by having warmed up all your breathing muscles, so they perform better.

Who Shouldn't Do This Exercise? Anyone who becomes dizzy easily from deep breathing, or who has ever passed out from deep breathing, shouldn't do this exercise without expert supervision.

Complete Breath #2, Mahat Yoga Prānāyāma

Prerequisite   Experience with breathing into each of the three sections of your lungs, diaphragmatic, intercostal, and clavicular.

Preparation   Assume the thunderbolt pose, vajra āsana [4.9, or with props, 4.10–4.12] or sit in a chair [4.13]. Relax in this pose, and sense your weight passing down through your body into the floor. Place you hands as you did in Complete Breath #1, your right hand centered on your lower lungs and your left hand centered on your middle lungs. Rest your elbows by your sides. Close your eyes [4.20].

The Exercise   Inhale in three parts, as follows: First exhale completely. Start filling your lower lungs, under your right hand, mostly filling downward so your belly puffs out; without a pause fill your middle lungs, under your left hand, expanding out to all sides; then fill your upper lungs, expanding to all sides as well as upward. You must *move your focus* from section to section to get the breath to move in this pattern. Fill your lungs with awareness and the air will follow.

Exhale in three parts, as follows: Start emptying from your lower lungs, under your right hand; continue without pause, emptying from your middle lungs, under your left hand; then continue emptying from your upper lungs, squeezing all the air out until you are empty. Repeat, inhaling and exhaling in this pattern.

Remember to get a *C* for effort. Breathe lazily. If you start feeling short of air or tense, stop for a few breaths and then try it again. If you can't make it feel comfortable after several tries, discontinue the practice.

To Finish   After twenty breaths or five to seven minutes, give up all your breathing effort. Rest your hands on your thighs, letting your breath do whatever it wants to. In about two minutes, stretch and lie down in the corpse pose. Rest there for another three to five minutes.

Benefits   They are the same as for Complete Breath #1. The sitting posture makes you more alert so your mind wanders less. This makes the practice more potent, increasing the benefits.

Who Shouldn't Do This Practice? Anyone who becomes dizzy easily from deep breathing, or who has ever passed out from deep breathing, shouldn't do this exercise without expert supervision. Also, anyone who, after three or four attempts to do the complete breath, still finds it tension-producing or uncomfortable should discontinue the practice and seek instruction from an experienced teacher.

How to Sequence the Sectional Breath Practices

You can do the practices in the order given, or you can do them in this order:

Breathe into each of the three lung sections plus the complete breath, in the order given, *using only the corpse pose* or the modified corpse pose [4.2 and 4.3].

Or pactice all four breaths in the order given *sitting in the thunderbolt pose*, vajra āsana [4.9, or with props, 4.10–4.12] or sitting in a chair [4.13]. When you are finished, lie in the corpse pose with your eyes closed for three to five minutes, simply relaxing, breathing automatically.

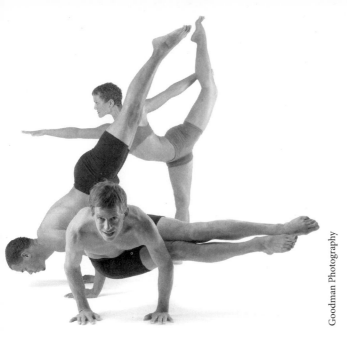

Goodman Photography

5

Postures, Āsanas

Tantra Yoga and Hatha Yoga view your body as an extension of your mind. Put another way, if you change something about your body, you change your mind as well. Since Yoga's main goal is to refine your mental capacity so you can see who you are and what the world really is all about, Tantra Yoga and Hatha Yoga focus on your body as well as your mind, training your body as *a way to train your mind*. This concept of traditional Yoga has survived in most of the modern Yoga systems. One can find it reflected in many statements by modern Yoga writers. Box 5.1 contains a sampling.

The Benefits of Practicing Yoga Poses

Yoga poses (āsanas, pronounced ah-sa-nas) function in traditional Hatha Yoga as a rung on a ladder to somewhere else. The ladder of Hatha Yoga techniques and disciplines leads to refined awareness, and ultimately if one continues long enough and arduously enough, to awareness that sees beyond the ordinary filters through which most of us look at

reality. That state of clear seeing is called samādhi (see Box 1.1, "Meditation Defined"), and it is the goal of all traditional Hatha Yoga āsana practice.

Yet many people practice Yoga poses for the fitness or health benefit they provide. Āsanas' benefits are so noteworthy that the U.S. National Institutes of Health (NIH), which is the principal government research agency concerned with medical science and health, has devoted part of its budget to researching the health benefits of Yoga āsanas and breathing.[1]

The benefits of Yoga āsanas result from the ways the various poses use your muscles, joints, breath, and mind (in the form of mental focus). Let's look at these elements of Yoga poses so we may understand better how they improve your health.

[1] The division of the NIH concerned with Yoga is called the National Center for Complementary and Alternative Medicine (NCCAM). Clinical studies funded by NCCAM have included: Iyengar yoga for young people with rheumatoid arthritis;
Evaluation of Yoga for chronic low back pain; Prenatal depression and a Yoga intervention; Meditation and exercise for prevention of acute respiratory infection;
Yoga for women attempting smoking cessation; Effectiveness of Integral Yoga on objective and subjective menopausal hot flashes.
Source: NCCAM web site, http://nccam.nih.gov, or call 1-888-644-6226

BOX **5.1**

Modern Yogins on Training the Body

Āsanas may appear to deal with the physical body alone but, in fact, different āsanas can affect the chemical messages sent to and from the brain and improve and stabilize your mental state. Yoga's unique ability to soothe the nerves, the medium between the physiological body and the psychological body, calms the brain, makes the mind fresh and tranquil, and relaxes the entire body.[2]

—B.K.S. Iyengar, Poona, India

Hatha yoga practice with its vast repertoire of movement expressions provides us with a veritable jungle gym to watch our reaction and responses to difficulty and challenge. Can we stay anchored in the silent mind regardless of where we find ourselves? What makes yoga yoga and not merely stretching or calisthenics is this mindful embodiment.[3]

—Donna Farhi, Christchurch, New Zealand

Āsana brings us completely into the present moment. With the practice of āsana we become aware of what is, of what sensations exist right now in the body and the corresponding thoughts that exist in the mind. This becoming aware of what is puts us in touch with emotions that may have been ignored or denied. When we are stretching the leg with awareness, that sensation of stretching brings us into the present moment. This coming into the present moment over and over again with the practice of āsana, either in a class or at home, creates a habit of awareness. This cognitive habit is meditative and can be emotionally therapeutic.[4]

—Judith Lasater, PhD, San Francisco, California

Muscles and Joints

Āsanas are physical exercises that engage your muscles and joints, the hinges of your skeleton. They are therefore called musculoskeletal exercises. The average body contains approximately 600 muscles, which constitute about 50% of the body's weight. About 40% of your body weight is composed of skeletal muscle, that is, muscles that move you, that you can feel and control. The other 10% of your muscle weight is internal organ muscles, like your heart muscle and the muscles around your blood vessels, bronchial tubes, and intestines, which in most cases you can't feel, and which you can't control. Obviously, any system of body transformation, whether the goal is power and stamina, capacity to relax, or ability to focus mentally, would need to focus on muscles. Yoga āsanas do just that.

Strength and Extensibility: Healthy Muscles

When one practices a variety of Yoga poses in one session, one usually vigorously contracts muscles and also elongates muscles to their maximum length. Contracting a muscle intensely

[2] Iyengar, *Yoga, the Path to Holistic Health*, 42.

[3] Farhi, *Yoga Mind, Body and Spirit*, 78–79.

[4] Feuerstein and Bodian, *Living Yoga: A Comprehensive Guide for Daily Life*, 43.

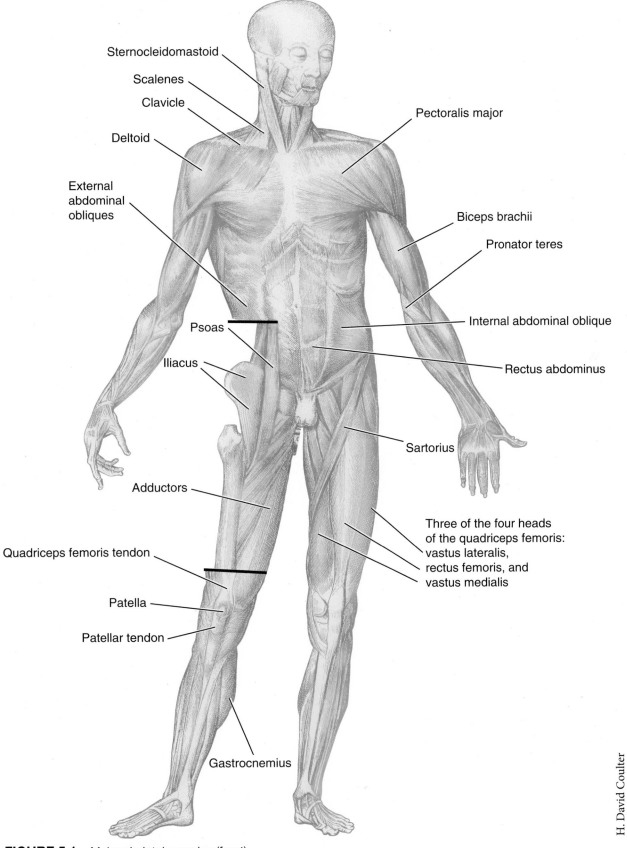

FIGURE 5.1   Major skeletal muscles (front).

Sternocleidomastoid

Scalenes

Clavicle

Deltoid

External abdominal obliques

Pectoralis major

Biceps brachii

Pronator teres

Internal abdominal oblique

Psoas

Iliacus

Rectus abdominus

Sartorius

Adductors

Three of the four heads of the quadriceps femoris: vastus lateralis, rectus femoris, and vastus medialis

Quadriceps femoris tendon

Patella

Patellar tendon

Gastrocnemius

H. David Coulter

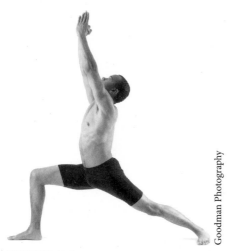

Goodman Photography

PHOTO 5.1   The warrior I pose is an example of an āsana that strengthens many muscles while also exercising your heart and respiratory system.

over and over strengthens it; elongating a muscle over and over makes it more extensible, increasing your flexibility. These two, strength and extensibility, are the properties of healthy muscles. (This is called "toned"[5] muscles.) Muscles that are strong are not optimally healthy unless they are extensible. Such muscles restrict the movement of joints and are prone to injury, such as tears in the muscles themselves, as well as in the tendons. Likewise, muscles that are very extensible but are not strong are not healthy either. Your joints controlled by these muscles will be unstable and prone to nerve compression and dislocation-type injuries. Most Yoga āsana sequences balance the two capacities of strength and extensibility. A good example of this is the sequence called "the salutation to the sun," taught on page 122 at the end of this chapter.

You can enjoy many benefits from regularly practicing Yoga poses that improve your muscle health:

Improved breathing

Stronger heart, better blood circulation

Stronger bones

Stronger attachments of ligaments and tendons to your bones

Improved balance

Improved range of motion

If your Yoga pose practice is aerobic—that is, it increases your heart and breath rate substantially for at least 20 minutes—and you do it three or more times per week, additional benefits include those that

are the benefits of any regular aerobic exercise regimen:

Slightly lower blood pressure

Faster metabolism, increased burning of calories

Increased sensitivity to insulin, a benefit to diabetics

Enhanced clot-dissolving substances in the blood, providing some prevention of strokes and heart attacks

Longer lifespan

Cardiovascular Benefits

When you use your muscles intensely, such as when you hold the warrior I pose [5.1], you demand more effort from your heart to circulate your blood to your hard-working muscles. And you demand more effort from your lungs to bring your muscles fresh oxygen and to remove carbon dioxide. This is called cardiovascular effort. Done consistently, such effort improves the health of your entire system.

Feelings and Relaxation

Healthy muscles, ones that are both strong and extensible, have more feeling and sensation because the nerves and nerve endings in your muscles are stimulated along with your circulatory and respiratory systems. This effect is obvious when you are exercising a muscle: you can feel it working or feel it stretching. But the increase in feeling lasts long after you stop exercising. If your body's most important muscle groups are toned you can feel more sensation throughout your body.

This capacity to sense your body produces a physical benefit: you can feel when you are tense or relaxed. You can feel when you are tired, when you are becoming stressed or anxious, or when you are starting to get sick. This can be a big advantage,

_____
[5] This word, tone, is somewhat confusing because it is widely used, with a variety of definitions. The dictionary defines tone as "a) The condition of an organism, organ, or part with reference to its normal, healthy functioning; b) the normal tension, or resistance to stretch, of a healthy muscle, independent of that caused by voluntary innervation; tonus" (Webster's *New World Dictionary*). This second definition corresponds to "muscle elasticity" which means the capacity of a muscle to return to its resting length after being stretched.

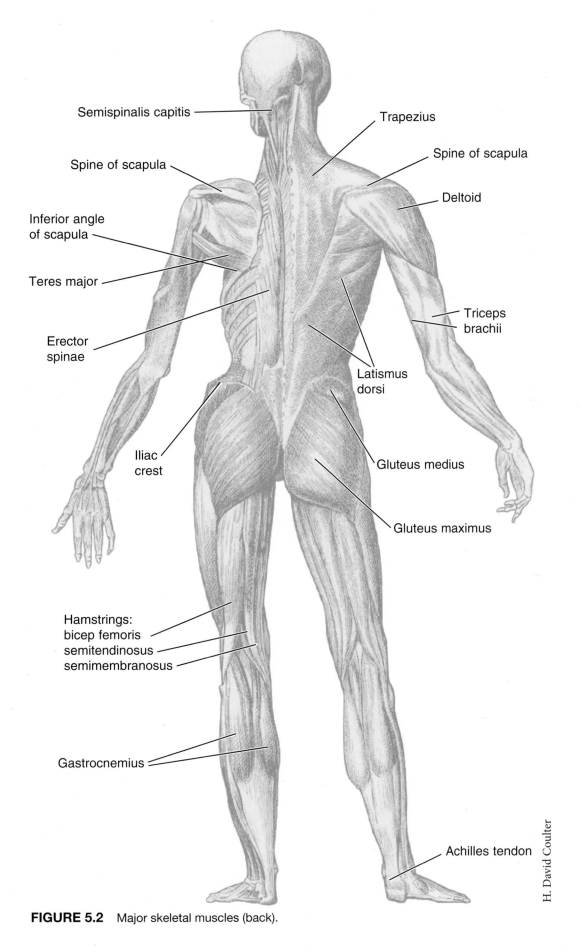

FIGURE 5.2 Major skeletal muscles (back).

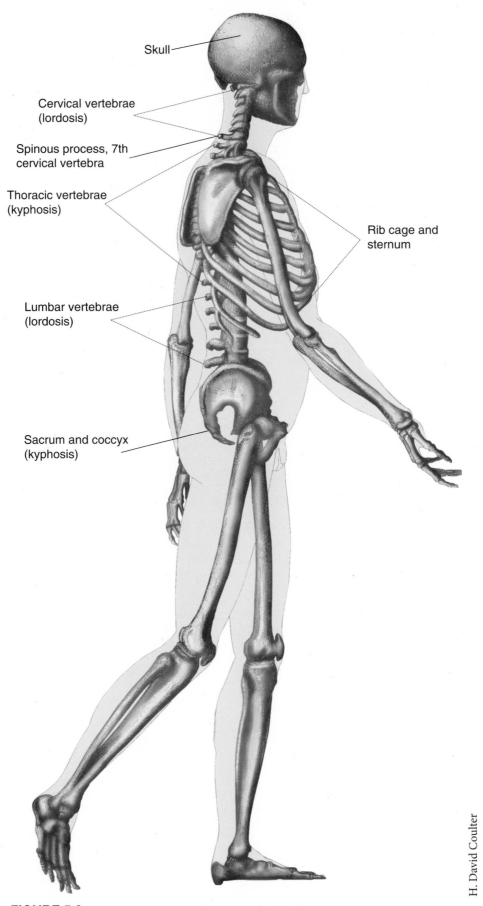

Skull

Cervical vertebrae
(lordosis)

Spinous process, 7th
cervical vertebra

Thoracic vertebrae
(kyphosis)

Rib cage and
sternum

Lumbar vertebrae
(lordosis)

Sacrum and coccyx
(kyphosis)

H. David Coulter

FIGURE 5.3   The skeleton and the regions of the spine.

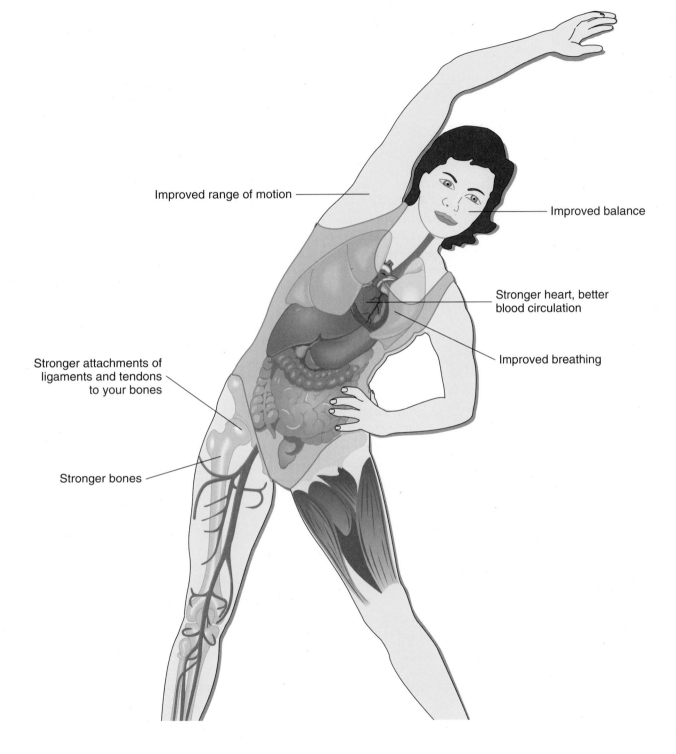

Improved range of motion

Improved balance

Stronger heart, better blood circulation

Improved breathing

Stronger attachments of ligaments and tendons to your bones

Stronger bones

FIGURE 5.4   Benefits of developing muscle tone with Yoga poses.

From *An Invitation to Fitness & Wellness,* 1/e, by Dianne Hales. Copyright (c) 2001 Wadsworth, a division of Cengage Learning, Inc.

because you can only do something to remedy your stress or imminent illness if you know about it. Some people are so numb to their feelings that they only learn that they are highly stressed when they hear from a doctor that they have an ulcer or they start to get bad headaches. What can you do if you are aware that you are stressed or getting sick? You can choose stress-reducing activities over stress-producing ones. You can get more sleep. You can do more Yoga exercises for stress reduction and for relaxation. And as you learn to sense yourself more often, you can relax the parts of your body that you habitually tense up, such as your shoulders or your lower jaw.

Feeling Emotions

Your capacity to sense your body, which is enhanced by Yoga poses, also helps you feel more of your emotions. As Judith Lasater states at the beginning of this chapter, "With the practice of āsana we become aware of what is, of what sensations exist right now in the body and the corresponding thoughts that exist in the mind. This becoming aware of what is puts us in touch with emotions that may have been ignored or denied."[6]

When you feel more of your emotions, you make healthier choices for yourself. You'll choose more fulfilling relationships. You'll choose more enjoyable jobs. You will learn more from your mistakes, from your choices that turned out badly.

Here's an example: you'll feel the excitement in your chest when you hear that your brother got the job he had worked so hard for. You'll feel the anxiety in your belly when you learn that you'll have to do a presentation in class. You'll feel the thick dullness in your arms and queasiness in your diaphragm when a friend tells you,

without making eye contact, that she has other plans, and you suspect she is lying. When these feelings arise again months later with some other (or the same) person, you'll remember the last time you felt them, and how the situation turned out. This sensory memory will help you make healthier choices.

Emotions function in us as the "juice," like electrical juice, that makes us feel alive and connects us to other people and to the world in which we live. In contrast, living in our minds and thoughts, without feeling in our bodies, feels dead, flat, and lonely. When a person who lives in her mind is asked, "How do you feel about me?" she might say, "Let me think about that." A person who is more in touch with her body might answer, "I like you," or "I am uncomfortable around you," or she might pause and sense her chest and belly so as to notice her feelings more clearly. Yoga āsana practice that enlivens and relaxes your muscles increases your "juice," and thus your ability to feel your emotions, even strong emotions like rage. In this regard, Yoga overlaps with the goals of psychotherapy.

Alexander Lowen, MD, an important pioneer in the field of body-centered psychotherapy, writes, "Therapy is a process of extending self-awareness . . . which is the ability to contain and sustain strong feelings. Bodily tensions and rigidity have to be gradually reduced so that the body can tolerate the higher level of excitation associated with strong feelings.[7]

Many Hatha Yoga practices, as you read in Chapter 3, work on changing the vital energy flows (prāna) in your body. The main way the yogin controls and stimulates prāna is with breathing practices. But āsanas are another important way to control and stimulate prāna. This energy is that which rushes through you when you

---

[6] Feuerestein and Bodian, *Living Yoga: A Comprehensive Guide,* 43.

[7] Lowen, *Narcissism: Denial of the True Self,* 61.

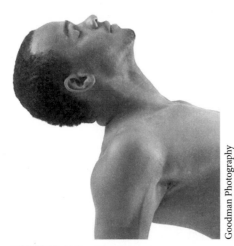

Goodman Photography

PHOTO 5.2 Pay attention to your sensations and your emotions when you practice yoga poses.

feel an emotion, like joy, sadness, or anger [5.2]. This is why your "body of prāna," your prāna-maya-kosha, is sometimes called your "emotional body." (See Chapter 3, "The Energy Body and the Five Bodies," page 38.)

A student of mine wrote about her experience with emotions while practicing āsanas and other Hatha Yoga practices over a weekend:

> One predominant experience of myself this weekend is noticing how strong an aversion to sensing and feeling there is within me. The programming that there is something so unforgivably wrong, not to mention hideous, with me seems so ingrained that the feeling seems to stay with me even when I consciously resist it. This weekend I saw that wrongness and ugliness as just another mechanism, albeit a powerful one, that keeps me from true feeling and perceiving. In effect, it says, "It is not a good idea to be with yourself because it would only bring up disappointment, your being so inadequate and all." This workshop gave me the opportunity to stop running so much from myself.

Relaxation

Another important benefit of using your muscles in āsana practice is reduction of tension, renewal of energy, and lessening of stress. Here's why this happens. When you gently stretch a muscle, it relaxes.

This is especially true if the muscle has first been warmed up by contracting it repeatedly. You've probably had a cramp in your calf muscle that you relieved by pulling back on your toes so your ankle flexed. This is the same principle. If you properly stretch a majority of your skeletal muscles, as often happens in an hour-long yoga class, you will feel relaxed. Relaxed muscles use up less oxygen, discharge less carbon dioxide, and use up less glycogen (sugar), resulting in your feeling more energetic. Relaxed muscles also allow more blood to circulate through them. In contrast, when you hold your muscles tense, you use energy, restrict blood flow, and get tired sooner.

Much of this tensing up is unconscious. It is a habit. But when your well-stretched body starts to feel more alive and relaxed, you will also feel more clearly your habitual tension when it returns after your Yoga class, as it inevitably does. This new awareness is a huge help because it enables you to do something about it. You can consciously relax a muscle if you can feel that you are tensing it.

Try this exercise. Close your eyes and sense your shoulders. Just feel whatever you notice in your shoulders and in the muscles all around them. Do this for a minute or two.

Did you instinctively relax your shoulders? Or did you instinctively tighten them? Most people relax them. We naturally relax tense muscles because it feels good. Tension is uncomfortable.[8]

When your muscles are well-toned with Yoga āsanas, you feel more sensation and emotion, you have more energy, and you are more relaxed. You can break bad habits, like keeping your legs tense all the time, and you can make healthier choices with the new information you have.

Mental Focus

Since the ultimate goal of Yoga poses is maximum awareness of who you are and your place in the universe, all of Yoga's intermediate goals are concerned with increasing awareness. You accomplish this by focusing your attention when you practice Yoga āsanas—and every other Yoga practice, for that matter. You pay attention

---

[8] Ornstein and Sobel, *Healthy Pleasures*, 3.

Safety Guidelines

- If you are unwell or have a chronic health condition, consult a physician before starting a Yoga āsana practice.
- Stay in touch with your sensations.
- Keep breathing; refrain from holding your breath.
- Stop or change what you are doing if you feel pain or strain.
- Practice where it is warm and well ventilated.
- Practice on an empty stomach, or at least 2 hours after a meal.
- Try easy poses first, harder ones later. When doing harder poses, or more intense stretches, do an easy version of the pose first.
- Take it easy, get a *C* for effort, relax in the midst of doing, and yet practice your Yoga poses with precision.

to what you are doing and what you are feeling. When you increase your ability to sense yourself and become more deeply in touch with what you are really feeling, you can do this many times throughout the day. This is an important component of psychological health.

Guidelines for Practicing Yoga Poses

Safety

Focus on your sensations when you do Yoga poses. This helps you avoid injuring yourself. The key to safe

practice is to avoid pain and strain [5.3]. Contrary to what you might have heard, pain is not a requirement when one is building strength and when one is stretching. In fact, it is counterproductive! Not only can you easily injure yourself, but you also slow down your progress toward strength and limberness.[9]

Be gentle with your legs, your back, and your hips. Keep part of your attention on the areas of your body that you are relaxing, even while other areas are exerting. I call this "doing and not-doing." It is expressed in the *Yoga Sutra*, 2.47, when Patanjali states that posture (āsana) must be performed while relaxing all effort, so that there is no agitation in the body.[10]

Keep your focus on *your* body and *your* sensations. If you look around the room at other people during class, or if you feel competitive with others in the class, or with your teacher, you lose touch with your own sensations and your own limits. Then you are much more likely to pull a muscle or tendon, or tear a ligament.

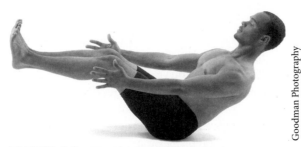

Goodman Photography

PHOTO 5.3 The key to safe practice is to avoid pain and strain by modifying a pose to suit your strength and flexibility. For example, here is an easier way to do the boat pose, nava āsana: perform it with bent knees.

---

[9] Ornstein and Sobel, *Healthy Pleasures*, 105.

[10] Feuerstein, *The Shambhala Encyclopedia of Yoga*, 268.

Breath in the Performance of Poses

Breathing is easy. If you let yourself be, you will breathe well and naturally. That is the trick when doing Yoga poses. The "get a C for effort" idea is especially useful for breathing in a pose. Using your muscles will naturally make you breathe more deeply. Let it happen. Many poses will naturally increase your breath in certain parts of your lungs. Let it happen. Slowing down your movements will naturally slow down your breath. Let it happen.

Your breath always moves you, undulates you, like waves rocking a boat. Let it happen.

I recommend that you leave your throat relaxed when practicing poses. Also relax your belly as much as possible so it can puff out on your in breath, allowing for a diaphragmatic breath (see Chapter 4, "Benefits of Diaphragmatic Breath," page 61). Leave the floor of your pelvis muscles (pubococcygeal muscles) relaxed, as well as your lower jaw and your face. Avoid holding your breath. If you catch yourself holding your breath, reduce your effort and let your breath flow again. You may experience your breath pausing or stopping at the top of the inhalation or at the bottom of the exhalation. That's OK.

Once you have familiarized yourself with natural easy breathing in Yoga poses, you can learn to coordinate your breath with your movements. For example, you may discover that you naturally inhale when you bend back or lift a limb, or exhale when you bend forward or lower a limb [5.4]. This kind of breathing works best and is easiest when you have completed the breath practices that you learned in Chapter 4. The specific breath patterns that accompany āsanas are best learned from a teacher, although you can learn a lot from your own experience.

The next stage of working with breath-focused movements is to concentrate *mainly* on your breathing, and to allow the movements to be initiated by the breath. Your arms inhale over your head and grow longer. Your torso exhales down toward your legs and releases into the pull of gravity. When you move this way, your movements tend to accommodate deeper and smoother breathing, without effort. When this happens, you may begin to feel the increasing flow of energy, prāna, in your body.

Slowing Down, Going Nowhere, Paying More Attention

Āsana practice is like a meditation. The point is to be there, to do and to feel the pose. The point isn't to fix yourself, to change yourself, or to accomplish something. Take time to draw your awareness inward before you start moving into a pose. After you come out of a pose, stop in the neutral or rest position and sense yourself. This interim time is actually the most important for deepening and expanding awareness. Be curious. Ask, "How did that āsana make me feel?"

Parasympathetic Nervous System

Practicing āsanas as described in these guidelines settles you into your parasympathetic nervous system, your

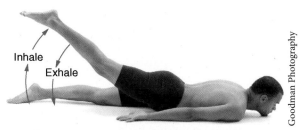

Inhale
Exhale

PHOTO 5.4 Once you have familiarized yourself with natural easy breathing in Yoga poses, you can learn to coordinate your breath with your movements.

Goodman Photography

> ## BOX 5.3
>
> # Movement Vocabulary: Flex and Extend
>
> When you move a joint so that you are creating a sharper angle, such as when you bend your elbow, it is *called flexion*. When you straighten a joint, it is called *extension*.
>
> In the case of your spine, the terms are less obvious. When you bend forward, such as when you reach down to tie your shoes, you *flex* your spine. When you bend in the opposite direction, as if you were reaching toward the ceiling to unscrew a light bulb in a ceiling fixture, you *extend* your spine. When applied to spinal movements, extend doesn't mean "to lengthen." For that, I will use the terms *reach* or *lengthen*.
>
> For other joint movements I will use common words such as *twist* and *side bend,* instead of technical terms such as *rotation, medial rotation, lateral rotation,* and *lateral flexion*.
>
> When you are lying on your back on the floor it is called "supine," and when you are lying on your stomach it is called "prone."

calm, unworried, "I-can-handle-it" nervous system. (See Chapter 4, "Effects on Your Nervous System," page 61.) Your muscles, lungs, and heart work more efficiently when you are operating from the parasympathetic nervous system. You have more stamina, your digestion works better, you feel less stress, and your mind is more open to sensations and to insights. In short, you experience more of the benefits of Yoga. And those benefits last longer.

Using Props

The use of props—blocks, belts, blankets, bolsters, chairs, and special benches—are a recent innovation in Yoga. They were developed by B.K.S. Iyengar in Puna, India, and by his students (see Chapter 8, "Choosing a Yoga Style or Lineage," page 156). Iyengar has greatly influenced modern Yoga methods, so props are used in many Yoga classes. Many other Yoga lineages do not use props.

If your instructor teaches poses with the aid of props, you will find them a useful addition to the practice. If your teacher does not use props, I think you will find that Yoga poses can be adjusted to your body in many ways. Because of these variations in Yoga classes, and since this book is written for use with every style of Yoga, I present poses here without the use of props, except in a few cases where a pillow or blanket is used.

The Poses of Hatha Yoga

I have grouped fifty poses into five broad categories to make it easy to find them in the book: lying-down poses, sitting poses, standing poses, inversions, and the salutation to the sun series. I present them in the order in which they can be practiced, balancing one kind of movement with another. (See Box 5.5, "The Key to Balanced Stretching: Spinal Range of Motion (ROM)," page 85.) The poses can also be combined in many other sequences. A usual āsana class will contain poses from several or all of these groups.

How Many Repetitions Should I Do?

This is very personal. I suggest you repeat each pose the minimum number given here to start with. If you feel fine and unstrained after that, do a few more. Each day the pose will feel a little different, and you may do a different number of repetitions. This approach gives you the opportunity to ask your body, "Another?" Listen and feel your muscles' and bones' answer.

Lying Down Poses

These can be done on a sticky mat (a plastic or rubber Yoga mat), on a thick blanket, on a rug, or on a thin cotton-batting-style Yoga mat.

Corpse Pose (Shava-Āsana) \sha-vah-sa-na\

Preparation   Lie supine on your mat [5.5]

The Exercise   Position your arms next to your sides, palms up or down, shoulders dropped away from your ears. Place your legs close together, heels touching if possible, but let your toes drop apart as your relaxed legs turn out a little. Your lower back should be close to the floor. If you can easily slide your flat hand under your lower back, then move your tailbone toward your feet so that your pelvis tilts your lower back closer to the floor. If your chin juts up and your neck tips

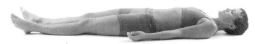

PHOTO 5.5

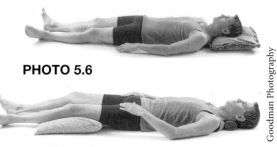

PHOTO 5.6

PHOTO 5.7

back, put a pillow or folded blanket under your head so that your neck is comfortable [5.6]. Relax your whole body feeling the places where you press into the floor and relaxing there. Surrender your weight to the floor.

To Finish   Roll onto your side or stomach before you sit up.

Benefits   This is the pose you will use for most relaxation practices, which might involve additional breathing or concentration instructions. All by itself, this pose is very relaxing.

Cautions/Adjustments   If your back, neck, or shoulders hurt or are uncomfortable in this pose, you can make them more comfortable with one or more of these adjustments: place your hands on your upper thighs or hips with your elbows resting on the floor. You can also place a rolled up hand towel under your neck to gently support its arch, and place a pillow or a folded blanket under your knees to elevate them slightly [5.7].

Pelvic Tilt in Modified Corpse Pose, Shava-Āsana

This is the same exercise as Diaphragmatic Breath #2 in Chapter 4, page 58, in which you tilt your pelvis so that you flatten your lower back toward the floor as you exhale and let your pelvis tip back to neutral as you inhale, which slightly arches your lower back upward (1/2 to 1 inch) to

Goodman Photography

its usual resting position [5.8–5.9]. Do about ten repetitions, or until you feel noticeably more relaxed.

Modified Supine Holding Big Toe Pose I (Supta Pādāngustha Āsana) /soop-ta pah-dahng-goost ah-sa-na/

Preparation   Start in corpse pose.

The Exercise   Draw your right knee up toward your chest, clasping it with your hands interlaced. Reach away through your left leg, out through your heel, flexing your ankle [5.10]. Try to keep this leg on the floor as you pull gently downward on your bent leg, further flexing your knee and hip and tucking your thigh toward your chest. Hold for three breaths, sending your breath into your right flexed hip joint. Straighten your right leg back to the floor, and repeat with other side. Then do the whole cycle once or twice more.

To Finish   Return to corpse pose.

Benefits   Relaxes and stretches your lower back (lumbar spine). Warms up your hip joint and stretches the muscles in your buttocks.

Modified Supine Holding Big Toe Pose II (Supta Pādāngustha Āsana)

Preparation   Start in corpse pose.

The Exercise   Draw both knees toward your chest and clasp your hands together around them, interlacing your fingers, hugging your thighs in toward your chest [5.11]. Feel the stretch in your lower back. Breathe against your lower back and against the floor, massaging your lumbar spine from the inside with your breath. Continue for five to ten breaths.

To Finish   Release your legs and straighten them along the floor. Take an inventory of your sensations in the corpse pose.

Benefits   This is an excellent exercise for lower backache. It relaxes and stretches the lower erector muscles of your back. The diaphragmatic breath that is induced by this pose relaxes you and massages your abdominal organs and colon, helping with digestion and elimination.

Cautions/Adjustments   Heavier people or pregnant women may want to create space between their thighs and pull their knees individually with each hand toward their chests. This is also a good variation for anyone [5.12].

Bound Bridge Pose I (Sethu Bandha Āsana) \set-hu bund ah-sa-na\

Preparation   This pose is best done on a non-skid surface like a Yoga mat. From the corpse pose, bend your knees and place your feet on the floor near or against your buttocks, hip-width apart, arms alongside your trunk, palms down.

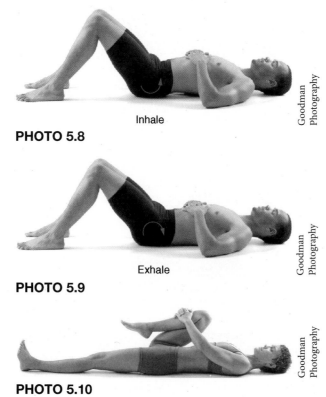

Inhale

PHOTO 5.8

Exhale

PHOTO 5.9

PHOTO 5.10

Goodman Photography

Goodman Photography

Goodman Photography

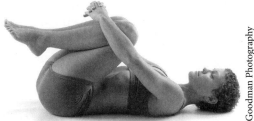

PHOTO 5.11

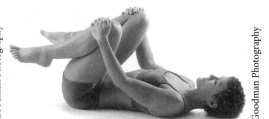

PHOTO 5.12

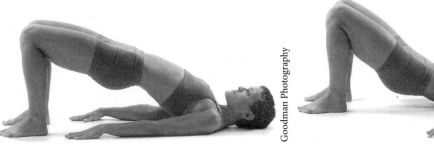

PHOTO 5.13

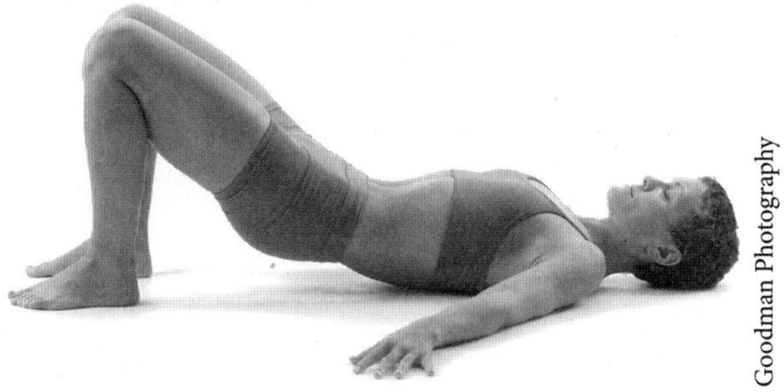

PHOTO 5.14

The Exercise   Inhale and press down through your feet and raise your pelvis and all of your mid and lower back off the floor as high as you can without strain or pain. Simultaneously press down with your arms and hands to support your lift, and squeeze your tailbone in [5.13]. Exhale and lower your back toward the floor by lowering your upper spine little-by-little, vertebra-by-vertebra [5.14], until you have rolled your whole spine back onto the floor. Repeat this five to seven times.

Next, hold the pose with moderately deep breathing. Draw your shoulder blades closer together, and squeeze your thighs toward each other as if you had a ball between your knees. Your knees stay hip-width apart.

To Finish   Exhale and roll your spine back onto the floor. Straighten your legs into the corpse pose. Rest.

Benefits   This pose strengthens your thighs, erector muscles, and abdominals. It stretches your abdominal muscles and lower intercostal muscles, stimulates diaphragmatic breath, and massages your abdominal organs.

It is a safe way to fully extend your lower spine.

Cautions/Adjustments   Please don't strain to go higher than is reasonable for you. Any amount of elevation of your pelvis is effective in this pose.

Bound Bridge Pose II, Sethu Bandha Āsana

Preparation   Attain bound bridge I.

The Exercise   Bend your elbows and turn your hands so your fingers aim away from your spine. Rise onto your tiptoes and work your hands under your pelvis as shown, keeping your elbows close together. Rest some or all of your weight into your hands. Drop the soles of your feet to the floor [5.15]. Lift your sternum up and draw your shoulder blades together and deep into your back. You can straighten your legs somewhat to intensify the pose [5.16].

To Finish   Support your bridge with your legs and back muscles, and bring your arms back to the floor. Then exhale as you lower your spine onto the floor. Straighten your legs into the corpse pose. Rest.

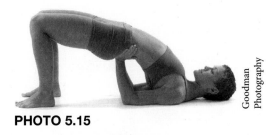

PHOTO 5.15

Goodman Photography

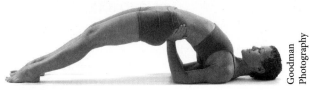

PHOTO 5.16

Goodman Photography

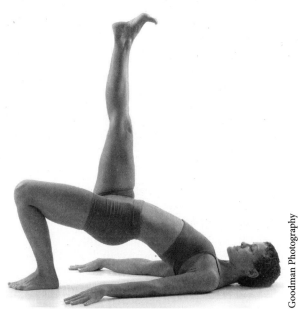

PHOTO 5.17

Goodman Photography

The Exercise   Once you have attained bound bridge II, raise one leg to vertical (or as high as you can raise it), with your ankle flexed, reaching up along the back of your leg and out through your heel. Lift your sternum up and draw your shoulder blades together and deep into your back [5.17]. Press firmly into the floor with your supporting foot. Hold for a few breaths. Lower your leg beside the other and repeat on the other side.

To Finish   Same as for bound bridge I and II.

Benefits   This pose contracts your muscles more intensely because your weight is supported by only one leg. It stretches your hamstrings and iliopsoas, works your hip flexors, stimulates diaphragmatic breath, and energizes your pelvic region.

Cautions/Adjustments   You may need to practice the other bridges for a while to build strength for this pose. Do not strain to accomplish it.

Belly-Turning Pose (Jathara Parivartana Āsana) \jut-ha-ra pa-ri-var-tan ah-sa-na\

Preparation   In corpse pose, spread your arms sideways on the floor, palms down. Draw your knees up toward your chest, keeping them together [5.18].

The Exercise   Inhale in this position. Exhale as you tip your knees off to your right and in the direction of your extended arm, looking left and keeping your left shoulder blade on the floor. Twist only as far as is comfortable. Keep your knees together and drawn up toward your chest, your abdominal muscles slightly engaged [5.19]. Then inhale as you untwist, bringing your knees up to their starting position, your head returning to center. Exhale and twist to the other side in the same way [5.20]. Repeat this five to eight

Benefits   This pose provides all the benefits of bound bridge I, and adds a more intense abdominal stretch and more extreme extension of your lower back.

Cautions/Adjustments   If your pelvis doesn't get very high in bound bridge I, omit this pose. Come out of it right away if it hurts your back or wrists.

One-Legged Bound Bridge Pose (Eka Pāda Sethu Bandha Āsana) \ek-a pah-da set-hu bund ah-sa-na\

Preparation   Same as for bound bridge II.

The Key to Balanced Stretching: Spinal Range of Motion (ROM)

We have now moved our spines in the three most important ranges of motion—flexing, extending, and twisting. These movements both stretch and contract the major muscles that control your body's position in space. They also release energy in your body when you alternate flexion and extension of your spine. These motions not only tone your muscles, but they also wake you up! In addition to these three ranges of motion, your spine can bend laterally, that is, to the side. This action affects some muscles that are not worked by flexing, extending, and twisting, so it is an important movement to include in your practice of āsanas. (See sitting side bend pose [5.70] and side-angle pose [5.102].)

You will tone your core muscles most effectively if you incorporate the four ranges of motion—flexion, extension, twisting, and side bending—into your practice.

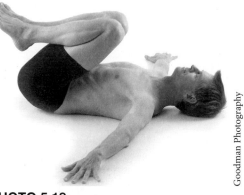

PHOTO 5.18

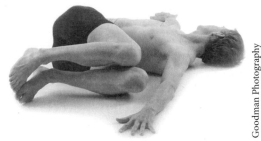

PHOTO 5.19

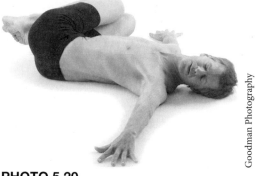

PHOTO 5.20

times on each side. Then do one more on each side, but hold the twist for thirty seconds to a minute.

To Finish   Return to center with an inhalation. Exhale and drop your feet to the floor and slide them away to return to the corpse pose.

Benefits   The belly-turning pose is wonderful for your lower back. It stimulates diaphragmatic breathing, so it massages your organs.

Cautions/Adjustments   If your range of motion is limited, place pillows or blocks on either side of you into which you can rest the weight of your legs as you twist [5.21]. Do this cautiously if you have had any spinal disc injuries.

Upward-Facing Back Stretch (Ūrdhva Mukha Paschimottana Āsana)\ *oordh-va* **mook-ha pas-chi-mo-tan ah-sa-na**\

Preparation   From the corpse pose, draw your knees up toward your chest, keeping them close together. Clasp your toes with your arms on the outside of your legs. If you can't

Goodman Photography

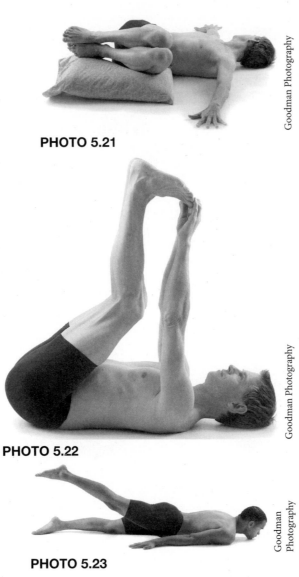

PHOTO 5.21

PHOTO 5.22

PHOTO 5.23

reach your toes, clasp your lower legs near your ankles or at your calves.

The Exercise Straighten your legs, keeping hold of your toes (or ankles), but don't straighten them all the way, at least at first [5.22]. Let gravity hold your whole back against the floor, keeping your head resting on the floor. Keep the back of your neck long. Maintain the straightening effort in your legs with slightly deeper-than-normal breathing, sending your breath toward the place in your back where you feel the stretch. You may feel more stretch in the backs of your legs, so feel that too, but bring much of your awareness to your sensations in your lower back, which is the main

focus of this pose. Hold this, continuing to extend your legs, for about ten breaths, or longer.

To Finish Bend your knees, still holding your toes. Then release your toes and lower your feet to the floor. Rest there for a few breaths. Then straighten your legs into the corpse pose.

Benefits This pose stretches your hamstring muscles along the backs of your legs, your gluteus muscles in your buttocks, and especially your lower-back muscles. Like the poses above, it encourages diaphragmatic breathing. It also increases the circulation in your legs.

Cautions/Adjustments The amount of bend in your knees is personal. Anyone who can catch their toes can do an effective stretch here. Straighter knees are not "better." If your head comes off the floor or your neck bends back uncomfortably, place a pillow under your head before you start.

Half Locust Pose (Ardha Shalabh Āsana) \ahr-dha sha-labh ah-sa-na\

Preparation From the corpse pose, reach your left arm over your head along the floor and roll over your left side onto your stomach (prone). Lie with your chin on the floor and your arms at your sides, palms up. This is the prone corpse pose.

The Exercise Reach out through your right leg, pointing your toe, press your arms and hands (palms down) into the floor, and slowly raise your leg off the floor, keeping it straight [5.23]. Raise it as high as it will go without strain. Then lower it slowly to the floor, still reaching out though your leg and toes. Release it completely. Immediately reach out through your left leg and raise and lower it in the same fashion. If you are comfortable using your breath along

Goodman Photography

Goodman Photography

Goodman Photography

with movement, you can inhale as you lift your leg, exhale as you lower it. Repeat about five times on each side.

To Finish End in the prone corpse, releasing your head to one side. Relax into the floor with automatic breathing.

Benefits Strengthens numerous important muscles in your legs and torso while it stretches others. A very safe hip extension exercise.

Cautions/Adjustments If your leg won't rise, just *engage the muscles* that *try* to raise it, holding these muscles engaged for a few seconds. Then slowly release them, *as if* you were raising and lowering your leg. As you gain strength and flexibility you may find that your leg does rise in the half locust pose. If your back hurts when you attempt to lift your leg, discontinue the pose.

Full Locust Pose I, Pūrna Shalabh Āsana

Preparation Assume the prone corpse pose, your chin on your mat (not turned). Make fists and slide them under your pelvis either in a palms-downward position or in a palms-facing position. [5.24].

The Exercise Start an inhalation with your diaphragm and press down through your fists and arms. Reach out through your legs and feet, toes pointing, and engage your muscles to raise both your legs off the floor [5.25]. Raise them as high as they will go, keeping them fairly straight. This takes a lot of effort. If you experience pain at any point stop immediately and rest. If your legs don't rise, just engage the muscles that *try to* raise them. Exhale as you slowly lower your legs to the floor. Repeat this two to five times.

To Finish Bring your hands out from under your pelvis, resting your arms along your sides, and turn your head to one side. Rest.

Benefits Intense strengthening of extensor muscles of your hips, as well as lower back extensors. The full locust also strengthens your arms and shoulders. It stretches the front of your body and effectively extends your lower spine.

Cautions/Adjustments Engage your muscles *gradually* to raise your legs. *Do not* hold your breath or jerk your legs up. If your neck is uncomfortable with your chin on the floor, you can instead tuck your chin toward your chest and place your forehead on the floor. If neither of these makes the pose do-able, lie on an elevated surface, like a folded thick blanket, with your head extending off the end of the blanket [5.24]. Hold this pose only if instructed to by a Yoga teacher. *Do not do this pose* if you have spinal disc problems or injuries.

Full Locust Pose II, Pūrna Shalabh Āsana

Preparation Lie prone, arms by your sides, palms up, chin (or forehead) on the floor.

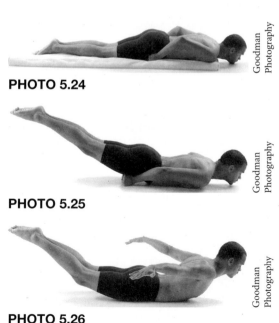

PHOTO 5.24

PHOTO 5.25

PHOTO 5.26

Goodman Photography

The Exercise   Inhale and lengthen both your legs and your spine, reaching from both directions, upward and downward. Simultaneously raise your legs *and torso* off the floor, and raise your arms beside you horizontally, reaching toward your feet. Gaze upwards, slightly tipping your head back [5.26]. Then exhale as you lower your torso and legs to the floor. Relax completely for an instant, softening all your weight into the floor; then repeat the exercise. Do two to five repetitions.

To Finish   Relax prone with your head turned to one side, arms down along your sides.

Benefits   Same as those for full locust I, plus more strengthening and stretching of muscles in your upper back, chest, and neck.

Cautions/Adjustments   See full locust I, above. This pose can be done with your arms raised over your head (this takes more effort), or with your hands clasped behind your head and your elbows spread, in which case it is called the leviathan, *makarāsana* (ma-kar-ah-sa-na).

Cobra Pose, (Bhujunga Āsana) *bhoo-jung-gah-sa-na*\

Preparation   Lie prone, with your hands on the floor under your shoulders [5.27], your toes pointed, your eyes closed.

The Exercise   Exhale, then inhale as you lengthen your spine and raise your head and chest, while you also reach out through your legs and feet. [5.28] Use your torso muscles to achieve your lift, not your arms and hands. Your hands simply rest on the floor. Exhale and descend to the floor. Repeat three to five times, inhaling as your rise, exhaling as you lower. This is the warm-up to the cobra pose. For the full cobra, add hand pressure to your lift, pushing your torso and head higher, while increasing the curve in your upper spine. Hug your shoulder blades into your back as you do this and keep your elbows near your sides. Also keep your pelvis on the floor. [5.29] Inhale as you rise into the pose, exhale as you descend back to the floor. Relax for an instant, then repeat. Do three to five repetitions of the cobra, then hold the lifted pose with deep breathing. While holding it, reach out through your legs and feet, keeping the tops of your feet on the floor. And reach out through your spine and neck, creating as much curve as feels good to you.

To Finish   Exhale as you lower your torso and chin to the floor. Rest for five to ten breaths.

Benefits   Stretches your abdominal muscles, enhances mid-chest breathing, and calms your nervous system. This pose fully extends your whole spine, especially your lower back.

Cautions/Adjustments   Refrain from straightening your arms, even if you

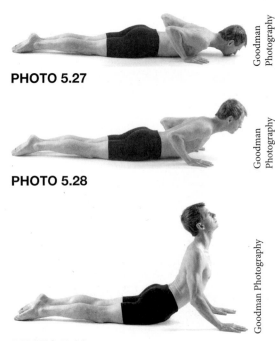

PHOTO 5.27

PHOTO 5.28

PHOTO 5.29

Goodman Photography

are quite limber. Instead, focus on lengthening your spine, from your pelvis up through your neck, and reach out through the top of your head. Avoid tipping your head too far back. Continue to lengthen the back of your neck even as you extend it.

Four-Footed Staff Pose* (Chaturānga Danda Āsana) *\cha-toor-ang-ga dund ah-sa-na

Preparation From prone position, place your hands under your shoulders and flex your ankles to put the balls of your feet on the floor.

The Exercise Inhale, then exhale as you press downward with your feet and hands to lift your body two to six inches off the floor, staying straight. Keep your buttocks in line with the rest of your body. Keep your neck in line with your spine, so your face is looking downward [5.30]. Hold this with deep breathing, feeling the effort in your muscles. Return to the floor after five to fifteen seconds. Repeat two to three times. If you lack the arm strength for this lift, perform it with your knees on the floor as shown in 5.31.

Goodman Photography

PHOTO 5.30

Goodman Photography

PHOTO 5.31

Goodman Photography

PHOTO 5.32 Incorrect

Goodman Photography

PHOTO 5.33

Goodman Photography

PHOTO 5.34

To Finish Relax in the prone corpse pose, with your head turned to the side.

Benefits The pose strengthens your abdominal muscles, arms, shoulders, and chest.

Cautions/Adjustments When doing the pose, engage your abdominal muscles and lengthen your lower back to keep from tipping your pelvis, which would raise your buttocks out of alignment [5.32].

Half Boat Pose* (Ardha Nāva Āsana) *\ahr-dha nahv ah-sa-na

Preparation In the prone corpse pose, raise your left arm overhead and roll via your left side onto your back, assuming the corpse pose. Place your hands on the floor beside your waist.

The Exercise Inhale. Then exhale and press down with your hands and raise your torso and your legs forty-five degrees until your feet are about the height of the top of your head. Lift your sternum, and look at your feet. It is easier if you bend your knees somewhat [5.33]. Reach your arms horizontally toward your legs at shoulder width, balancing on your buttocks and tailbone [5.34]. Hold this for five to eight deep breaths. Come down by replacing your hands on the floor under the small of your back, exhaling as you lower your feet to the floor by bending your knees, and then rolling your spine onto the

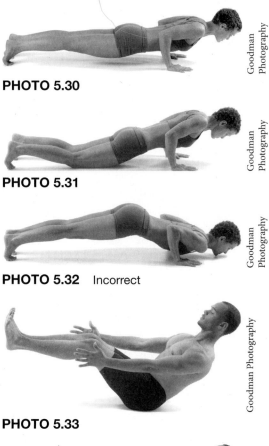

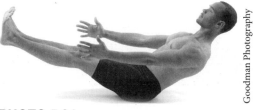

floor. Repeat two to three times. If you lose your balance, return to the floor for a short rest; then try it again.

To Finish   Rest in the corpse pose.

Benefits   The half boat improves your balance, increases your energy, and strengthens your abdominal muscles.

Cautions/Adjustments   If this pose is too uncomfortable for your tailbone, place more cushioning under your seat before you start. Extra cushioning also makes it easier to balance in the pose, as does bending your knees. Some students will need to strengthen their abdominal muscles

with other poses before they will be able to do the half boat. If the pose hurts your back, discontinue it.

Modified Supine Holding Big Toe Pose II, Supta Pādāngustha Āsana

This was taught earlier in this chapter, on page 82 [5.12].

Upward-Facing Back Stretch, Ūrdhva Mukha Paschimottana Āsana

This was taught earlier in this chapter, on pages 85–86 [5.22].

Upward Straightened Legs Pose (Ūrdhva Prasarita Pada Āsana) \oordh-va pra-sa-ree-ta pahd ah-sa-na\

Preparation   Lie in the corpse pose.

The Exercise   Draw your knees toward your chest and straighten your legs upward, flexing your ankles and reaching your whole back and head into the floor [5.35]. If your legs don't straighten all the way, just keep engaging the straightening effort [5.36]. Lower your legs by reversing the movement, bending your knees toward your chest, dropping your feet to the floor, and then extending your legs away along the floor to the corpse pose. Repeat the pose five to ten times. Inhale as you lift, and exhale as you lower your legs.

Now repeat the leg lift, but this time hold the pose with the legs vertical, or reaching toward vertical, feeling the dynamic of straightening your legs while flexing your ankles, extending up along the backs of your legs and out through your heels. It is OK to let your legs shake. Hold this for four to eight deep breaths.

To Finish   Use an exhalation to lower to the corpse pose. Rest for thirty seconds to one minute, focusing on your sensations.

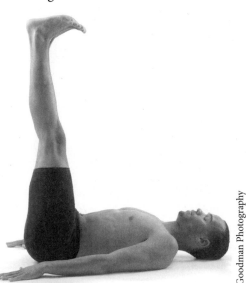

PHOTO 5.35

Goodman Photography

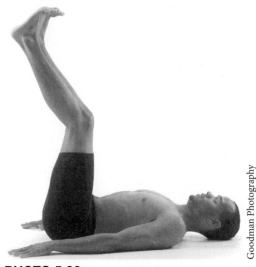

PHOTO 5.36

Goodman Photography

Benefits This pose strengthens your hip flexors and quadriceps (thigh) muscles, strengthens your abdominal muscles, stretches your calves and hamstrings, relaxes your lower back, and dramatically increases blood circulation in your legs.

Cautions/Adjustments You can practice this against the wall. Lie with your buttocks pressing the wall, your legs extending up the wall. This will enable you to hold the pose much longer, but with less strengthening effect.

Fish Pose I (Matsya Āsana) *maht-syah-sa-na*\

Preparation The corpse pose.

The Exercise Flex your ankles and straighten along the backs of your legs. Press your elbows and the back of your head into the floor to raise your chest upward, arching (extending) your spine [5.37]. Draw your elbows closer together, spread your fingers, and press your arms and hands (which can slip under your buttocks) into the floor to support your arching spine. Breathe deeply as you hold the pose, lengthening your spine by pressing into the floor with your buttocks and with the top or top-back of your head. Let your chest open as you lift the center of your chest to the ceiling. Hold this for five to eight deep breaths.

To Finish Carefully slide your head away from your body and lengthen your back along the floor, returning to the corpse pose.

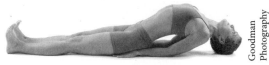

PHOTO 5.37

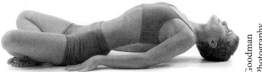

PHOTO 5.38

Benefits The fish pose lowers your blood pressure, stretches your chest muscles, extends your spine fully, and deepens your intercostal (middle) breathing.

Cautions/Adjustments Avoid tipping your head too far back in this pose. Think of lengthening your neck in a gentle curve.

Fish Pose II, Matsya Āsana

Preparation Cross your legs at the shins while lying on your back.

The Exercise Push up into the fish pose, as above, while reaching your knees apart and toward the floor [5.38].

To Finish Carefully slide your head away from your body and lengthen your back along the floor. Then straighten your legs to the corpse pose.

Benefits Same as for fish pose I, plus it opens the hips.

Cautions/Adjustments Same as for fish pose I.

Note: Both fish poses can also be done from a sitting position. The completed fish pose, *pūrna matsya āsana,* is presented on page 47.

Upward-Facing Back Stretch, Ūrdhva Mukha Paschimottana Āsana

This was taught earlier in this chapter, on page 86 (see Photo 5.22).

Upward-Facing Bow Pose (Ūrdhva Dhanur Āsana) *oordh-va dha-noor ah-sa-na*\

This pose is also called the half wheel pose (*ardha chakra āsana,* pronounced ahr-dha chuk-rah-sa-na). Practice this pose after you have

Goodman Photography

Goodman Photography

learned it in class. Your instructor can help you perform it properly and safely.

Preparation   From the corpse pose, bend your knees so your feet are on the floor close to your buttocks, hip width apart. Reach over your shoulders and place your hands on the floor with your fingers facing your feet [5.39].

The Exercise   Inhale and press into the floor with your hands and feet. Simultaneously raise your pelvis starting with your tailbone and moving toward your waist. Exhale, then inhale and press the back of your head and your hands into the floor and tip your head back as you raise your

chest, placing the top of your head between your hands [5.40]. Hold this pose with deep breathing, continuing to lift your pelvis and chest by pressing down with your hands and feet, and feeling your sensations. Hold for two to eight breaths. To come down, carefully slide your head away while pressing more strongly with your hands. Then lower your back to the floor starting with the upper, then middle, then lower back. Extend your arms and legs into the corpse pose and rest. Repeat once or twice more.

To Go Higher   When you repeat this pose, you could go into a more advanced version of it by pressing substantially harder with your hands and feet, raising your whole body off the floor into an arch, so that your head hangs between your arms [5.41]. This is an intermediate-level pose, requiring great arm strength and joint flexibility.

To Finish   Rest briefly in the corpse pose. Your back will likely feel uncomfortable because it needs a counter-pose (which comes next).

Benefits   This pose provides an intense extension for your spine; it stretches all the muscles in the front of your body and it strengthens your arms and legs.

Cautions/Adjustments   Do not do this pose if you have disc problems. Perform this pose on a non-skid surface like a rubber Yoga mat or hard floor. Do not strain your arms to attain this pose. Approach the more advanced pose carefully and do not do this pose if it hurts your wrists.

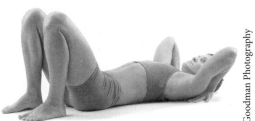

PHOTO 5.39

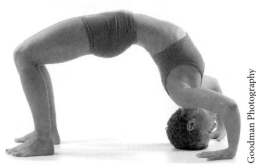

PHOTO 5.40

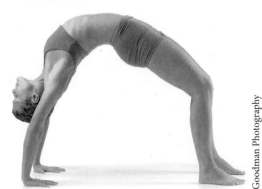

PHOTO 5.41

The Plow Pose (Hala Āsana) \hal-ah-sa-na\

Practice this pose after you have learned it in class. Your instructor can help you perform it properly and safely.

Goodman Photography

Preparation   Start in the corpse pose, lying on a folded blanket with your head off the end of the blanket. Do the upward straightened legs pose, urdhva prasarita pada āsana, found on page 90 [5.35 and 5.36].

The Exercise   Inhale fully. Exhale and simultaneously press your hands into the floor as you swing your legs over your head, raising your pelvis off the floor. Place your hands on your buttocks and push your pelvis up so that you roll onto your middle back, with legs extending over your head [5.42]. Now support your lower back with your hands and drop your knees toward your head with your legs straightening. Hold your legs parallel to the floor [5.43], or lower them until you can touch your toes to the floor over your head [5.44]. Hold the pose for four to twelve breaths.

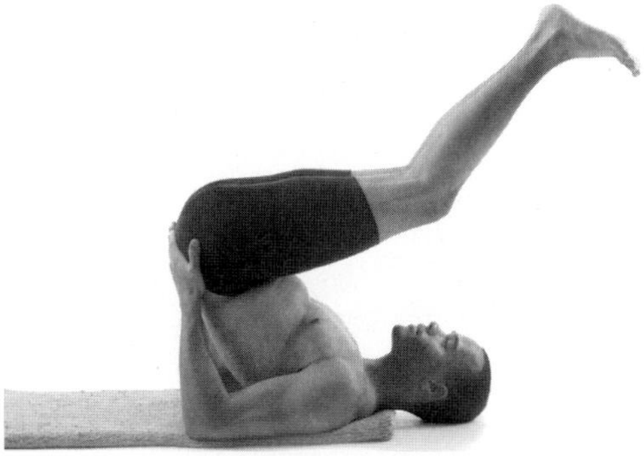

To Finish   Supporting your lower back with your hands, reverse the movement until your feet rest on the floor, your knees bent. Rest here for a few breaths. Then extend your legs into the corpse pose when you are ready to do the next pose.

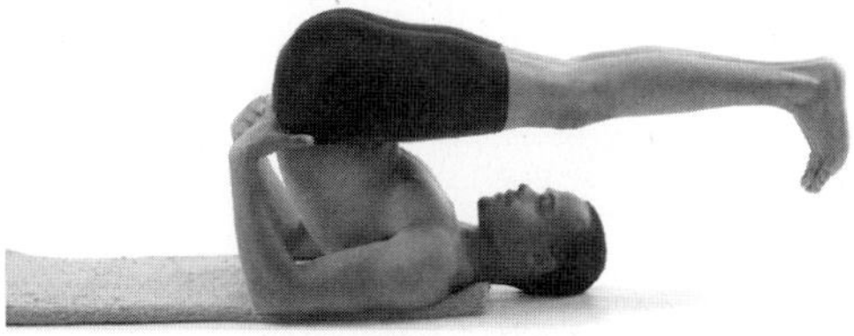

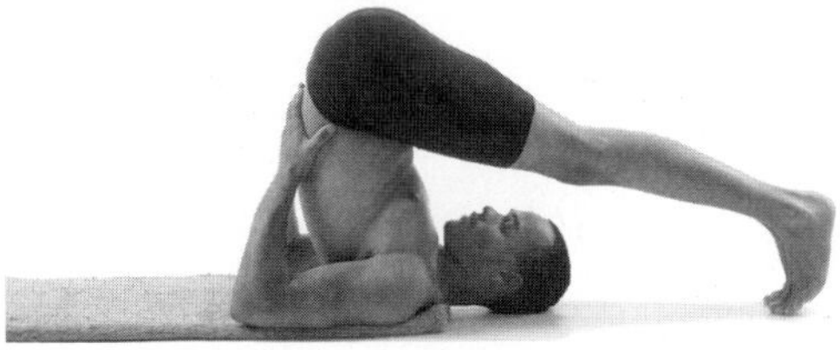

Benefits   The plow offers you the most thorough lower back/hamstring stretch of all the āsanas.

Cautions/Adjustments   This pose must be followed immediately with a counter-pose or your back is likely to hurt. Do not do this pose if you have disc problems.

Half Bow Pose (Ardha Dhanur Āsana) \ahr-dha dha-noor ah-sa-na\

Preparation   From corpse pose raise your left arm overhead and roll onto your belly. Lie prone with your arms along your sides, your chin on the mat.

The Exercise   Bend your right leg to bring your foot near to your right buttock. Reach back with your right hand and take hold around the top of your foot [5.45]. Pull on your foot as you contract your thigh muscle to extend your leg, thereby raising your torso and your thigh off the floor, with your foot/hand rising above you. Keep the hand of your left arm beside you on the floor, and keep your left foot on the floor [5.46]. Keep your pelvis and shoulders level; that is, don't twist your back. Lift your head and gaze up without crunching the back of your neck. Hold the pose for a few breaths, and then come down, lowering your chest, chin, and thigh to the floor and releasing your foot. Straighten your right leg and relax totally. Repeat on the other side. You can add a coordinated breath, inhaling as you rise into the pose and exhaling as you lower out of it. Do three to five repetitions on each side.

PHOTO 5.42

PHOTO 5.43

PHOTO 5.44

Goodman Photography

Goodman Photography

Goodman Photography

To Finish   Relax in the prone corpse pose, with your head turned to one side.

Benefits   The half bow is an excellent spinal extension; a good abdominal, chest, and shoulder stretch; and a strengthener for your erector muscles.

Cautions/Adjustments   Don't do the half bow if you have disc problems.

The Full Bow Pose (Dhanur Āsana) \dha-noor ah-sa-na\

Preparation   Same as for half bow pose.

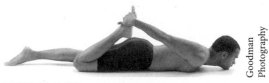

PHOTO 5.45

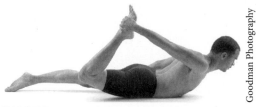

PHOTO 5.46

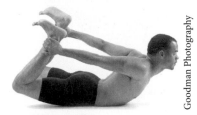

PHOTO 5.47

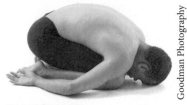

PHOTO 5.48

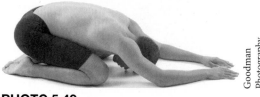

PHOTO 5.49

The Exercise   Bend both legs, catching around your feet where they meet your ankles (one at a time). Inhale and slowly raise your head and chest from the floor. On your next inhalation, pull against your feet with your hands and lift your thighs off the floor. Attempt to straighten your legs while pulling on your feet with your hands [5.47]. Hold the pose briefly with natural breathing; then reverse the sequence of movements to come down. Remain holding your feet and repeat once or twice more.

To Finish   Relax in the prone pose, your arms by your sides and your head turned to one side or centered.

Benefits   The bow massages your abdominal organs and intensely stretches your front torso muscles.

Cautions/Adjustments   Don't do this pose if you have liver or spleen problems, or if you have disc problems.

The Child Pose (Bala Āsana) \bahl-ah-sa-na\

Preparation   The prone corpse pose.

The Exercise   Rise onto your hands and knees, with your knees slightly apart. Sit back toward your heels as you lower your chest and head downward, letting gravity fold you. Rest your head on the floor, if it reaches it, your chest pressed against your thighs. Reach your hands back beside your feet, palms up, resting your elbows toward the floor [5.48], or extend you arms overhead, resting them on the floor [5.49] in the position called stretched child's pose (*utthita bala āsana,* pronounced oot-hi-ta ba-lah-sa-na). Hold this for one to three minutes, with natural autonomic breathing.

To Finish   Rise to your hands and knees. Then lie on your back in the corpse pose.

Goodman Photography

Benefits   The child pose is an effective and gentle stretch for your lower back, is calming to your nervous system, and is psychologically comforting.

Cautions/Adjustments   If the pose over-flexes your knees, place a pillow between your heels and your buttocks. If you are pregnant or overweight, create a space for your belly by allowing the knees to part slightly, as shown in Photo 5.49.

Belly-Turning Pose, Jathara Parivartana Āsana

This pose is taught earlier in the chapter, on pages 84–85 [5.19].

Modified Supine Holding Big Toe Pose II, Supta Pādāngustha Āsana

This pose is taught earlier in the chapter, on pages 82 [5.11].

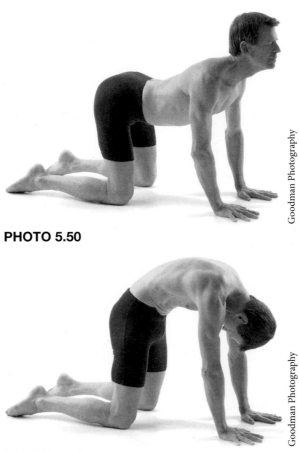

PHOTO 5.50

PHOTO 5.51

Corpse Pose, Shava-Āsana

This pose is taught earlier in the chapter, on page 81 [5.5]. Relax in this pose, focusing on your sensations of weight and of breath, for five minutes.

Sitting and Kneeling Poses

These can be done on a sticky mat (a plastic or rubber Yoga mat), on a thick blanket, on a rug, or on a thin cotton-batting-style Yoga mat.

Tiger Breathing (Vyagrah Prānāyāma) \vi-ah-grah prah-nah-yah-ma\

This two-pose sequence is also called cat-cow pose, marjarya āsana–bitila āsana, pronounced mah-jar-yah-sa-na and bi-ti-lah-sa-na

Preparation   Assume a four-footed pose on your mat. Your thighs and arms should be vertical, with your weight centered between them. Place your hands shoulder-width apart and your knees hip-width apart, and hang your head.

The Exercise   Inhale, slowly raising your head and sagging your middle back, tilting your pelvis to accentuate the extension of your spine [5.50]. Exhale, tilting your pelvis the other way, raising the middle of your back, creating an arch (flexing your spine), and dropping your head between your arms, chin reaching toward your chest [5.51]. Feel as if you are trying to reach your pubic bone to your forehead. Inhale, extending your spine and lifting your head. Exhale, arching your spine and lowering your head. Start each movement with your pelvis, which helps you start each breath with your diaphragm. Repeat five times focusing on your movement and muscle sensations, then five more focusing on your breathing,

Goodman Photography

Goodman Photography

guiding your movement with the flow of your breath.

To Finish   Exhale to your neutral, head-hanging starting position. Then sit back toward your heels, lowering your chest to your thighs in the child pose, bala āsana, taught earlier on pages 86–87 [5.48]. Rest here for a minute with effortless breathing.

Benefits   Tiger breathing is the best single Hatha Yoga exercise I know. It equally flexes and extends your spine while relieving gravity's effects on it. The breath-led movement massages your abdominal organs. The stretch in your back and chest opens your breathing, and your neck is wonderfully warmed up. Tiger breathing drops you into your parasympathetic nervous system because of your diaphragm's involvement (see page 52 in Chapter 4), and it clears your mind, slowing down your thoughts.

Cautions/Adjustments   Anyone can do this two-pose sequence. If you find coordinating the movement and breath confusing, dispense with the breathing instructions. If your wrists ache, make your hands into fists and place your knuckles against the floor so that your wrists are straight. Be sure to tilt your pelvis as far as it goes in each direction: your tailbone tucking under when you arch your back, your tailbone rising behind you as you sag your back.

The Cricket Action (Chiri Kriya) \chi-ree kree-ya\

Preparation   Assume a four-footed pose on your mat. Place your hands shoulder-width apart and your knees hip-width apart, and hang your head.

The Exercise   Inhale as you extend your right leg behind you with your toes staying lower than your hip while you extend your spine and raise your head. Near the end of your inhalation, raise your straightening leg as high as you can without twisting your back [5.52]. Exhale as you lower your lifted leg to horizontal, and then bend your knee all the way up toward your forehead, which is dropping toward your knee. Flex your spine [5.53]. Repeat five times on the right side, then switch sides during an inhalation. Do five more.

To Finish   End with an inhalation by returning to your all-fours starting position. Then sit back toward your heels, lowering your chest to your thighs in the stretched child pose, utthita bala āsana [5.49]. Let your breath become automatic and relaxed. Rest for a minute.

Benefits   The cricket action exercises your hip flexor and extensor muscles, as well as your whole spine, similarly to tiger breathing. Tiger breathing's other benefits also apply here.

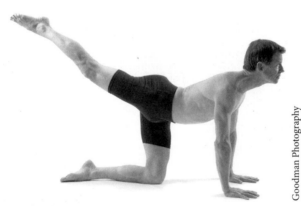

PHOTO 5.52

Goodman Photography

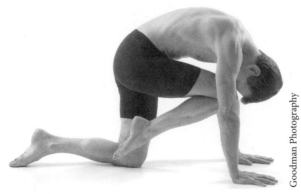

PHOTO 5.53

Goodman Photography

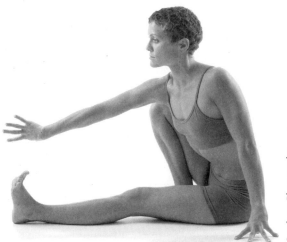

PHOTO 5.54

Goodman Photography

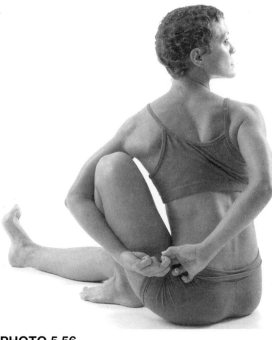

PHOTO 5.56

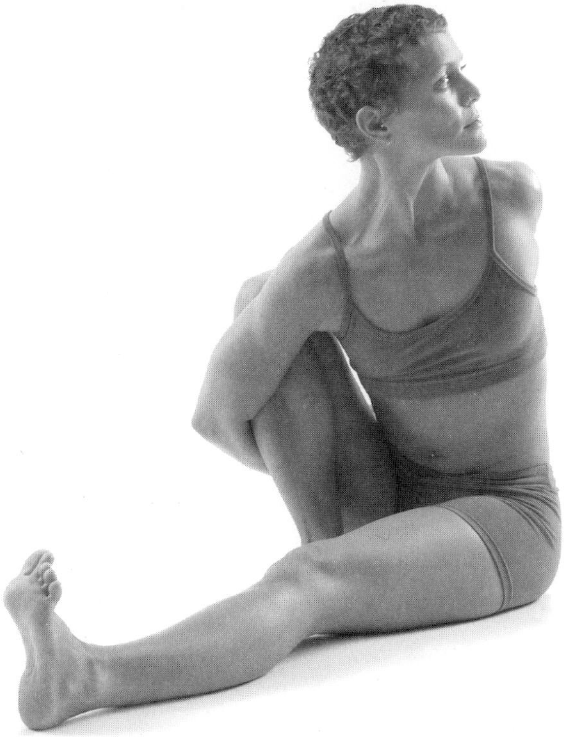

Goodman Photography

PHOTO 5.55

Goodman Photography

Cautions/Adjustments   Anyone can do this exercise. Be cautious if you have disc problems, especially during the leg lift. If your wrists hurt, make fists against the floor or place a partly rolled up Yoga mat under your palms.

The Sage Marichya Pose (Marīchya Āsana) \ma-reech-yah-sa-na\

Preparation   Sit with your legs extended, your spine upright, and your fingertips on the floor by your hips.

The Exercise   Bend your right leg and place your foot in front of your right groin. Turn toward your left and reach your right arm straight in front of you so it is directly over your straight left leg. Now lean forward and place your right shoulder just inside of your right knee. Rotate your right arm inward so that your palm faces to the right [5.54]. Wrap your arm around your leg and reach backward with your hand. Then reach with your left arm behind you and around, the back of your hand against your back, to catch the fingers of your other hand. Turn your head to the left while you use your arm loop to rotate your shoulders while straightening your spine [5.55]. Reach out through your straight left leg, flexing your ankle so your toes point up. Hold the pose, lengthening your spine up through the top of your head, with deep breathing for four to ten breaths. Repeat on the other side [5.56]. Then once more on each side, if you wish.

To Finish   Untwist and straighten your bent leg. Sit still with your eyes closed for thirty seconds, sensing your body.

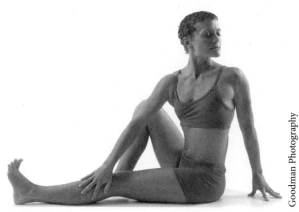

PHOTO 5.57

Goodman Photography

Benefits   The pose increases internal organ circulation by the compression-release effect of your diaphragm's fall and rise. It also releases tension from your spine and back muscles. And this, like many twists, stimulates diaphragmatic breathing, engaging your parasympathetic nervous system.

Cautions/Adjustments   If your hands don't come together behind you, place your right hand (with your right knee up) on your left lower leg, while your left hand is on the floor behind you. Use your arms to help you lengthen your spine and to twist, looking around to your left, behind you [5.57].

Head to the Knee Pose (Jānu Shīrsha Āsana)\jah-noo sheer-shah-sa-na\

Preparation   Sitting, legs extended, bend one leg so your foot's sole contacts your inner thigh, as close to your groin as you can, your knee dropping to the side. Place your palms together at your chest [5.58].

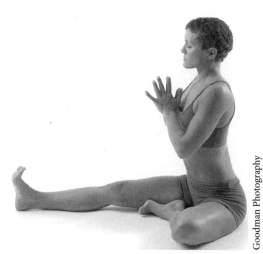

PHOTO 5.58

Goodman Photography

The Exercise   Inhale as you reach overhead, joining your hands and reaching upward through your spine and out the top of your head [5.59]. Exhale and lower your hands along the front of your body, reaching down your extended leg, bending forward from your hips, and taking hold of your leg wherever your hands reach. In order to allow your hips to tip forward, you may bend your extended leg, inclining your lower back toward your leg [5.60]. Your spine remains elongated, lengthening from your pelvis through your neck and head. Repeat, using your breath with the movement: inhaling as you rise and reach up, exhaling as you descend and bend forward. Repeat this movement three to five times and then hold the forward-bending pose with calm breathing.

In this pose, you might explore flexing your extended leg's ankle, and lengthen that leg by straightening your

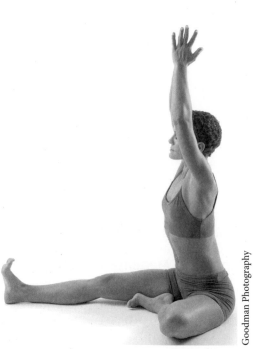

PHOTO 5.59

Goodman Photography

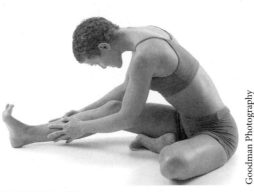

PHOTO 5.60

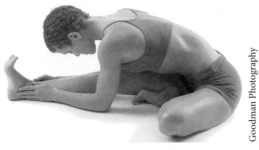

PHOTO 5.61

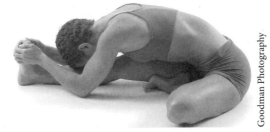

PHOTO 5.62

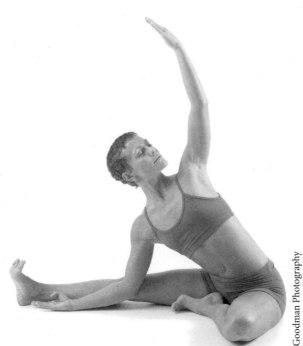

PHOTO 5.63

knee. Lengthen your torso, dropping your shoulders away from your ears, lengthening your neck [5.61]. The completed pose involves holding your foot and folding your torso to your leg so your head reaches your shin [5.62].

To Finish   Slowly rise to sitting erect, bringing your palms together in front of your chest [5.58]. Straighten your bent leg. Sit, legs extended, hands on thighs, and rest for thirty seconds.

Benefits   The pose provides an excellent spinal flexion and hamstring muscle stretch. It also strengthens your back's erector muscles.

Cautions/Adjustments   If your flexed knee hurts as you bend forward, reduce its bend, moving your foot further down your other leg. You could also place a folded blanket under your knee. Also, don't bend so far forward that it hurts. The restriction place in the pose may be your knee for a while. As you become more flexible (in your hips and back), this condition will likely change and you will be able to achieve more flexion in your spine.

Twisted Head-to-the-Knee Pose (Parivritta Jānu Shīrsha Āsana) \pa-ri-vrit-ta jah-noo sheer-shah-sa-na\

Preparation   Assume the head to the knee pose, with your right leg extended.

The Exercise   Slide your right hand and arm to the inside of your right leg and toward your foot as you reach overhead with your left arm and hand, your palm inward. Open your chest by drawing your left shoulder vertically over your right shoulder as you tip to the side, reaching your left arm upward strongly, but not beyond vertical. Simultaneously reach your right elbow toward the floor to the inside of your knee [5.63]. Push into the floor with both buttocks, rooting

100   Yoga for Fitness and Wellness

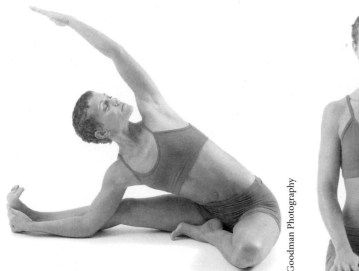

PHOTO 5.64

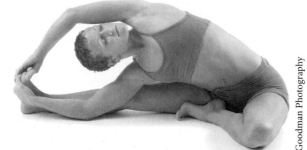

PHOTO 5.65

Goodman Photography

PHOTO 5.66

Goodman Photography

Benefits   This pose provides a side bend for your spine, an important range of motion that is under utilized in many series of āsanas. It also stretches your hamstrings and releases tension from your intercostal muscles, deepening your mid-lung breathing.

Cautions/Adjustments   "Farther down" is not "better." Keeping your alignment in this pose will benefit you more than will getting closer to your leg. Overstretching in this pose can injure your hamstring muscles.

Thunderbolt Pose (Vajra Āsana) \vah-jrah ah-sa-na\

Preparation   Fold a blanket in fourths to create a sitting pad, or use a couple of folded towels.

The Exercise   Kneel on the pad with your feet and knees together. Lower your buttocks toward your heels, letting your heels separate slightly, about six inches apart. Sit on your heels, resting your weight into your legs and feet. Sit erect so your back is in a position such as when you are standing. Adjust your buttocks on your heels so you can achieve this erect posture [5.66].

Close your eyes, relax your weight downward into the floor, and sense your breathing for thirty seconds to two minutes.

To Finish   Begin the next pose.

Benefits   The thunderbolt pose conditions your legs and hips for all other sitting poses. It extends your ankles and fully flexes your knees.

Cautions/Adjustments   If your knees hurt right away or after a short while in the position, place a pillow, folded blanket, or rolled up towel on top of your calves and feet, between

your seat to the floor, while you continue to straighten your right leg. In this pose you are lengthening your left side *and* lengthening your spine, from your tail bone up through the top of your head.

To increase the stretch, tilt further to your right, sliding your hand along your leg toward your foot and your elbow toward the floor. If you get that far, you can clasp your foot. Your shoulders remain vertically aligned and your left arm reaches out over your extended leg. Turn your head upward [5.64]. Breathe in the pose for one minute, then perform it on the other side.

If you are very flexible, clasp your foot with both hands while maintaining the vertical alignment of your shoulders [5.65].

To Finish   Sit comfortably erect, legs extended, and relax for thirty seconds.

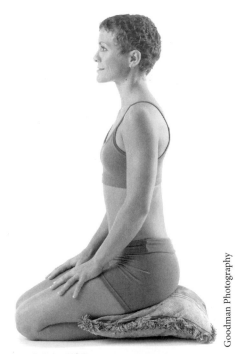

PHOTO 5.67

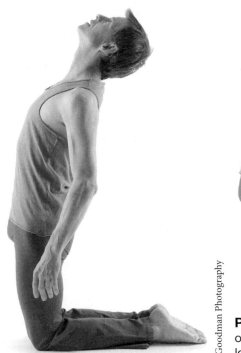

PHOTO 5.69

PHOTO 5.70 Incorrect. Note the over-extended neck and collapse in the lower back.

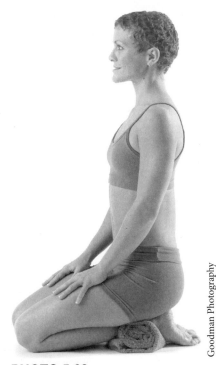

PHOTO 5.68

your buttocks and feet [5.67]. If your ankles hurt, place a rolled up towel or small pillow under your ankles [5.68]. If the pose continues to hurt your ankles or knees after you try it with pillows, omit it.

Incomplete Camel Pose (Sapūrna Ushtra Āsana) \sa-poor-na oosh-trah-sa-na\

Preparation Sit in the thunderbolt pose.

The Exercise Inhale, lean slightly forward, and rise to a kneeling position, spine erect, your arms hanging beside you. Push down through your knees and insteps into the floor and reach up through the top of your head, elongating your body (or so it will feel). Pause here for one or two breaths. Keep your pelvis over your knees as you inhale and lengthen your front, curving your spine in a slight extension (back bend), but *also lengthen your back as you* do this [5.69]. Tip your head back slightly, reaching out through the top of your head, letting your arms hang so that

your shoulders are pulled down by their weight. You are supporting your spine in this extension with your front and back torso muscles.

Do not thrust your pelvis forward as a way to achieve a curve in your spine [5.70]. Instead, lengthen your spine up and out of your pelvis as you anchor your knees and feet into the floor.

Don't hold your breath. Instead, as soon as you reach the camel pose, exhale and lift your torso to a straight position, your head rising up as if it were a helium balloon, then leaning slightly forward, sitting down on your heels in the thunderbolt pose. Repeat three to five times, inhaling as you rise all the way to the extended pose, exhaling as you return to the thunderbolt pose.

After you have done a number of repetitions, you may find that you can extend your spine more. You might *briefly* hold your breath in as you lengthen further into the extension. Follow your sensations and do this only if it feels good.

To Finish Rest in the thunderbolt pose.

The Importance of Caution in Upright Extensions (Back Bends)

The most dangerous of the back-bending poses are those where your spine is upright and bearing weight, such as in the camel pose [5.71]. The compression force in your intervertebral discs is amplified by bending, and that force is applied unevenly to the discs when you bend. This is as true of forward bending (flexion) as it is of back bending (extension), but flexion movements are more common to our bodies. Your muscles are more used to controlling them and are therefore stronger. This makes upright forward bends less dangerous than back bends, although if you have disc problems you should be cautious with both kinds of bends.

The keys to safe back bending (spinal extensions) are: Move slowly. Do not jerk or thrust your body into a pose. Strengthen your abdominal muscles and keep them strong, with poses like the pelvic tilt in modified corpse pose (p. 81), four-footed staff pose (p. 89), half boat pose (p. 89), upward straightened leg pose (p. 90), tiger breathing (p. 95), and cricket action (p. 96). Engage your abdominals in every upright spinal extension pose. Your abdominals link your pubic bone and the front of your rib cage, pulling your pelvis forward under the base of your ribs and tucking your tail-bone under.

Lift, lift, lift. When you lengthen your spine, the front of your body *and the back of your body* lengthen. This lengthening engages muscles that support your back. See the camel pose instructions for an example of this.

Don't go as far as you are able in upright extension poses until you are advanced at performing āsanas. There are lots of better (for beginners) extension poses that use a horizontal position, like the upward facing bow pose (p. 91) and the cobra pose (p. 88), which eliminate the compression force that occurs when you are upright.

Benefits   The camel increases diaphragmatic breath. It stretches your intercostal muscles, releasing chest tension and increasing mid-breath. It extends your spine, especially in your upper back (thoracic area).

Cautions/Adjustments   All upright extensions carry some danger for your lumbar spine. See Box 5.6.

Camel Pose (Ushtra Āsana) \oosh-trah-sa-na\

Note: you must be strong and quite flexible to even attempt this pose. Always warm up with the previous pose. I recommend that you do this pose only after learning it from a qualified teacher.

Preparation   Sit in the thunderbolt pose.

The Exercise   Inhale, leaning slightly forward and rising onto your knees. With your pelvis positioned over your knees (as in incomplete camel, above) breathe normally and extend your spine while lengthening your whole torso, both front and back, lengthening your spine up and out of your pelvis as you anchor your knees and feet into the floor. Lifting your sternum, catch your right heel with your right fingertips, then your left heel with your left fingertips. Realign your hips over your knees. Continue your spine's curve into your neck, so your head tips back, but not all the way [5.71]. Hold

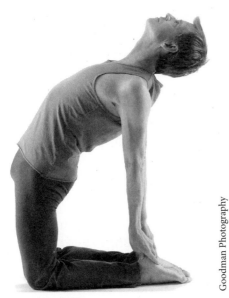

PHOTO 5.71

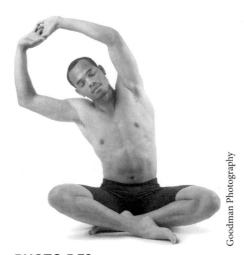

PHOTO 5.73

Goodman Photography

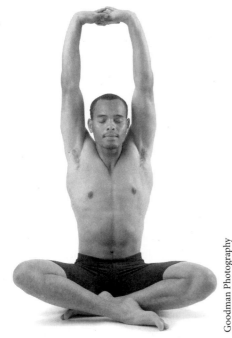

PHOTO 5.72

Goodman Photography

the pose with deep breathing for five to twenty seconds.

To Finish   Be careful coming out of the pose. If you have strong abdominal muscles, you can inhale and lift your torso to vertical, lengthening your spine all the way. Then sit down into the thunderbolt pose.

If you aren't sure of your strength, press down hard with your hands into your heels and lower your buttocks to your heels. Then rest in the thunderbolt pose.

Do not repeat this pose.

Benefits   This pose gives your spine a full extension, stretching your abdominal muscles to their maximum length. It increases abdominal breathing and opens your chest and heart region. It strengthens your breathing muscles if you breathe deeply while you hold the pose.

Cautions/Adjustments   You can perform the camel with flexed ankles, so your heels are higher and easier to reach. Also see Box 5.6 above.

Sitting Side Bend (Ūrdhva Baddha Hasta Sukha Āsana) \oordh-va bud-dha hasta sook-hah-sa-na\

This literally means "upward bound hands easy pose."

Preparation   Sit in a cross-legged pose, which is called easy pose, *sukha āsana* (sook-hah-sa-na), the leg position for which is shown in Photo 5.72. Interlace your fingers in front of you. Turn your hands outward so your thumbs point down and your palms face away from you. Raise your arms upward, straightening your elbows. Push down through your seat and reach up through your whole spine and through your arms, out through your palms [5.72].

The Exercise   On an inhalation, lengthen your right side so that your spine curves slightly toward your left, reaching out through the top of your head and your arms [5.73]. Do not twist; instead, keep your right shoulder over your left shoulder, not forward of it. Lower your shoulders away from your ears, sliding your shoulder blades down your back. Exhale as you return to upright, continuing to lower your shoulder blades down your back, still reaching up through your arms. Inhale and lengthen your left side and bend slightly toward your right. Repeat three times to each side.

To Finish   Lower your hands onto your knees and rest with eyes closed.

Benefits   Provides your spine with an essential range of motion, side bending. This stretches and strengthens your torso muscles, which hold you upright, helping you sit in meditative poses.

Cautions/Adjustments   If your hips are tight, you won't be able to bring your spine upright—your lower back will bow out to the back. To remedy this, elevate your buttocks by sitting on a meditation cushion or thickly folded blanket, so that your knees are lower when you cross your legs [5.74]. Don't worry if your arms incline forward at their

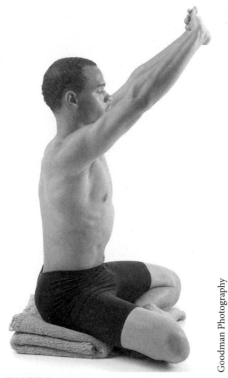

PHOTO 5.74

Goodman Photography

maximum lift position. Just keep lengthening them and drawing them upward.

Staff Pose (Danda Āsana) \dun-dah-sa-na\

Preparation   Sit with your legs extended, knees slightly bent, ankles flexed, toes pointing up.

The Exercise   Press your palms into the floor beside your hips, lengthen your spine upward, and position your shoulders over your hips. Drop your shoulders, sliding your shoulder blades down your back. Perch your head on top of your neck, directly over your shoulders. Some people must maintain bent legs to achieve this alignment [5.75]. Hold this pose with awareness and deep breathing, simultaneously reaching out through your legs and heels and also reaching up through your spine, out the top of your head. Hold for thirty seconds to one minute.

Only straighten your legs all the way [5.76] if you can do so without rocking back on your pelvis and without bowing out your lower back or leaning back.

To Finish   Progress to the next pose, the back stretch.

Benefits   The staff pose attunes your awareness to proper alignment in all other sitting poses. It strengthens your erector muscles.

Cautions/Adjustments   To make it easier, you may sit on the edge of a folded blanket so your seat is elevated higher than your legs, as shown in Photo 5.75. This also helps you straighten your legs.

Back Stretch (Paschimottana Āsana) \pas-chi-mo-tan-ah-sa-na\

Preparation   The staff pose, above.

The Exercise   Inhale as you tilt your spine forward without bending it. You may need to flex your knees more to achieve this. Then exhale and slide your hands down your legs as you bend forward from your hips, keeping your neck in line with your upper spine. Lengthen your whole torso, reaching out from the top of your head toward the space above your toes. Clasp your legs wherever your hands end up as you tip forward, and lower your shoulders away from your ears. Stay here for a few breaths; then with an exhalation, drop your head forward and bend down further to the limit of your stretch, perhaps sliding your hands further down your

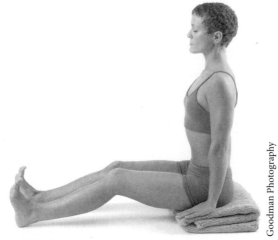

PHOTO 5.75   **PHOTO 5.76**

Goodman Photography

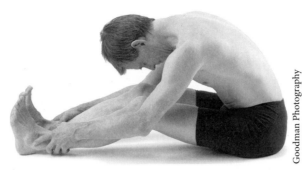

PHOTO 5.77

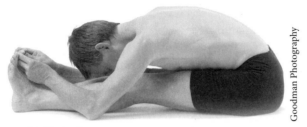

PHOTO 5.78

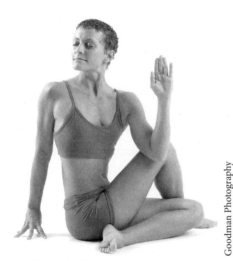

PHOTO 5.79

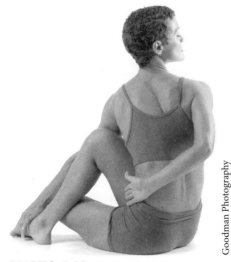

PHOTO 5.80

legs [5.77]. Rest your forehead on your legs if possible. You may now extend your legs more, to increase the stretch [5.78]. Hold this for thirty seconds to two minutes.

Stretching in this pose should feel intense and interesting, but not painful. If you would call your sensation "pain," back off by raising your torso a little, bending your knees more, or both.

To Finish Inhale to the staff pose from which you started. You may assist your back muscles in raising your torso weight by pressing down with your hands into your legs and walking them up your legs until you are sitting erect. Survey your sensations in this pose for a few breaths.

Benefits This produces a superb stretch for your lower back. It also stretches your hamstrings to their full length.

Cautions/Adjustments As with the staff pose, you may sit on the edge of a folded blanket so your seat is elevated higher than your legs.

Fish Pose, Matsya Āsana

This pose was taught earlier in the chapter, on page 91 [5.37 and 5.38].

Matsyendra's Half Spinal Twist (Ardha Matsyendra Āsana) \ar-dha mat-see-end-rah-sa-na

Matsyendra was a famous sage.

Preparation Sit in easy pose, sukha āsana, the easiest cross-legged sitting pose (see page 103).

The Exercise Raise your right knee so the sole of your right foot is next to your shin. Step this foot across your left leg so it is now on the floor by your thigh. Press both buttocks into the floor, although your pelvis may have to be slightly tipped. Twist to the right to reach your left arm to the outside of your right raised knee, with your shoulder close to your knee and your forearm and hand pointing upward. Place your right hand on the floor behind you and press down to lengthen your spine and to twist it. Turn your head to look over your right shoulder [5.79]. Hold this for three to ten breaths, continually lengthening and rotating your spine. Your breath will be very restricted. Keep it flowing; don't hold your breath.

In the more complete pose, catch your right ankle with your left hand, and reach your other arm (right) around behind you as far as it will go, with the back of your hand against your hip [5.80].

Repeat the pose on the other side.

To Finish Simply untwist your spine, unravel your legs, and sit in the easy cross-legged pose. Notice how deeply you breathe after your breathing has been so restricted in the twist pose.

Benefits This twist produces deeper diaphragmatic breath, releases tension in your spine and hips, and

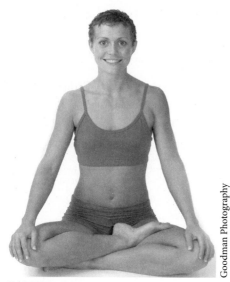

PHOTO 5.81

Goodman Photography

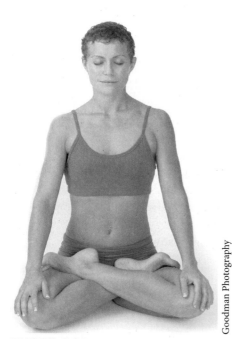

PHOTO 5.82

Goodman Photography

energizes you. The breathing against restriction produced by the pose massages your visceral organs, improving your digestion and elimination.

Cautions/Adjustments   Work up to this pose with simpler twists such as revolved belly pose (p. 86) and Marichya pose (p. 97). Even intermediate stages of this pose are effective. Attempt the pose described and stop wherever you reach your limits. Then hold that pose. You can't do it wrong. Any variation you come up with is fine. Most important, feel your body in your pose.

Half Lotus Pose (Ardha Padma Āsana) \ahr-dha pad-mah-sa-na\

Preparation   Sit in easy pose, sukha āsana (p. 103).

The Exercise   Bring your right heel in close to your groin, your knee opening out to the side, resting on or near the floor. Reach *under* your left shin and ankle with your fingers and lift your foot onto your upper right thigh, sole upward. Then straighten your spine and place your hands on your knees as shown [5.81]. Breathe slowly and deeply in and out five to ten times in this pose, relaxing more and more with each exhalation. Repeat this with your other foot on top.

To Finish   Reach under your ankle and slide it off of your thigh. Sit in the easy pose and sense your body with automatic breathing.

Benefits   This pose prepares you for meditation, which is the goal of all Hatha Yoga. So, in a way, your experience in this pose, and ones like it, is the goal of all the other poses.

Cautions/Adjustments   Try sitting on a meditation cushion or folded blanket at least four inches thick. *Do*

not force your leg up onto your thigh. You can seriously injure your knee. This pose is best learned from an experienced teacher.

The Lotus Pose (Padma Āsana) \pad-mah-sa-na\

This famous pose must be learned from a qualified Yoga teacher. I show it here to illustrate how the easy pose (sukha āsana) and half lotus pose (ardha padma āsana) are developmental stages leading to it. Don't despair if it looks impossible. Many yogins have achieved clear states of awareness without ever doing the lotus pose. *And* it is a great pose worth working toward. [5.82]

Corpse Pose, Shava-Āsana

Sense your weight and your breath in this pose for five minutes (p. 81).

Standing Poses

Mountain Pose (Tādā Āsana) \tah-dah-sa-na\

The Exercise   Stand with your feet hip width apart, parallel, toes spread out and on the floor. Evenly weight the corners of your feet by using this image: Imagine that your feet have four little legs in the four corners of the soles of your feet, and evenly weight these four legs. Your knees are straight but not locked back; relax your knees. (B.K.S. Iyengar suggests you contract your rectus femoris muscles, pulling up on your knee caps. I prefer a relaxed knee.) Position your spine so your pelvis is centered over your feet, your shoulders are centered over your pelvis, and your head is perched on top of your neck so it sits directly above your shoulders, with your gaze forward. Your arms hang relaxed at your sides with your hands relaxed [5.83].

Feel the forces that affect your body in this pose. First, feel the force pulling downward, gravity. Feel the weight of your head on your neck, the weight of your arms pulling down on your shoulders, and the weight of your upper body bearing down into your legs and finally into the floor through the soles of your feet. Second, feel the pressure of the floor pushing up against the soles of your feet. The floor isn't passive, as you may think, receiving your weight and not reacting to it. The floor is *pushing back up* into your feet with the same force with which your feet are pressing down into the floor. Feel this upward force in your legs and in your pelvis, then further up into your spine, all the way to the top of your head. This may feel to you like

a reaching-up feeling deep in your bones. It is the energy that holds you up. This upward-moving energy also enables you to feel when you are standing straight, with correct posture. See Photos 5.84 and 5.85 for examples of common standing postures that illustrate poor alignment.

To Finish   Wiggle your body and then stand normally. Explore this position by feeling the effect of the two forces (downward-moving and upward-moving) in your normal standing posture.

Benefits   You can discover whether you usually stand in a misaligned position by practicing the mountain pose. If you do, you probably walk and sit in such a position too. This is

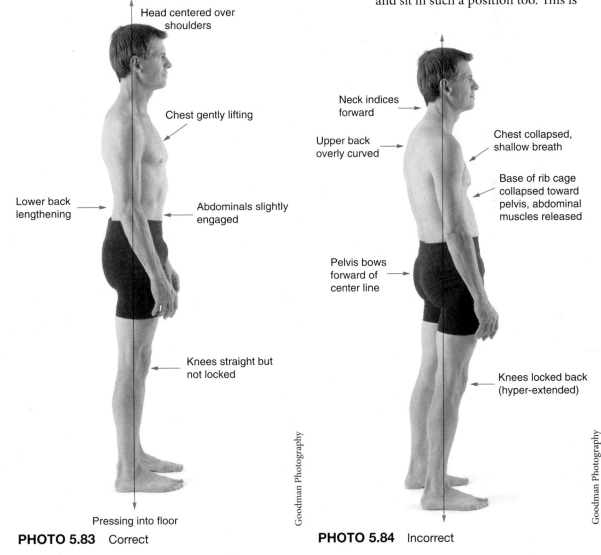

Reaching upward

Head centered over shoulders

Chest gently lifting

Lower back lengthening

Abdominals slightly engaged

Knees straight but not locked

Pressing into floor

PHOTO 5.83   Correct

Neck indices forward

Upper back overly curved

Chest collapsed, shallow breath

Base of rib cage collapsed toward pelvis, abdominal muscles released

Pelvis bows forward of center line

Knees locked back (hyper-extended)

PHOTO 5.84   Incorrect

Goodman Photography

Goodman Photography

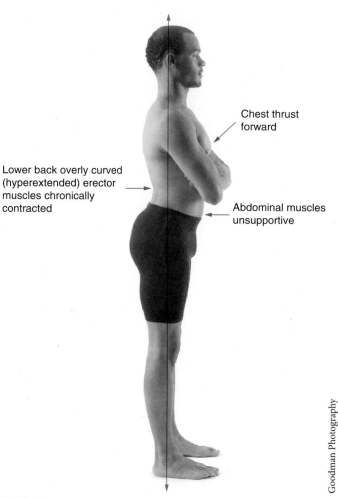

Chest thrust
forward

Lower back overly curved
(hyperextended) erector
muscles chronically
contracted

Abdominal muscles
unsupportive

Goodman Photography

PHOTO 5.85   Incorrect. Note the pelvis is behind the center line, and the shoulders are forward of it.

the first step in correcting your posture with Yoga āsanas.

Cautions/Adjustments   You will be better able to feel your legs and how they support you if you breathe with your diaphragm (p. 56). I recommend standing sideways to a full-length mirror too, so you can check your alignment.

Squat Pose I (Utkat Āsana) \oot-kat-ah-sa-na\

Preparation   Stand in the mountain pose [5.83].

The Exercise   Inhale deeply. Then exhale and bend your knees until your heels start to rise off the floor. Then straighten your knees slightly. Keep your torso as upright as you can,

balancing in the middle of your feet. Hold this pose with your arms reaching straight down [5.86]. Hold this pose for three to ten moderately deep breaths.

To Finish   Breathe in as you rise to standing straight again.

Benefits   The squat greatly strengthens your thigh muscles. It warms you up and increases your endurance.

Cautions/Adjustments   Don't stick your rear out in this pose. Instead, draw your pelvis forward under the base of your ribcage. Bend your knees only as far as you need to maintain this alignment; too much knee bend will force your pelvis to tip backward.

Squat Pose II, Utkat Āsana

Preparation   Stand in the mountain pose [5.83].

The Exercise   Inhale deeply. Then exhale and bend your knees until your heels start to rise off the floor. Then straighten your knees slightly. Keep your torso as upright as you can, balancing in the middle of your feet (avoid inclining your torso forward or backward). Hold this pose, raising your arms overhead with your palms joined, thumbs hooked together, drawing your arms back toward a position beside your ears [5.87]. Your arms may angle forward beside your cheeks. Simply maintain some effort to raise them higher. Hold this pose for three to ten deep breaths.

To Finish   Inhale as you rise to standing straight again, lowering your arms to your sides.

Benefits   The squat II greatly strengthens your thigh and back muscles. It warms you up and increases your endurance.

Cautions/Adjustments   Same as for squat I.

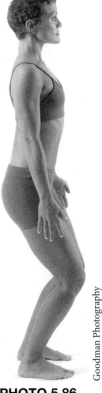

PHOTO 5.86

Goodman Photography

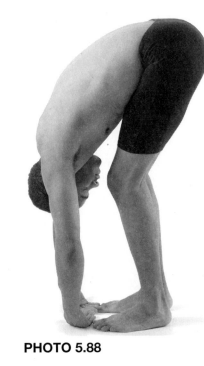

PHOTO 5.87

Goodman Photography

PHOTO 5.88

Goodman Photography

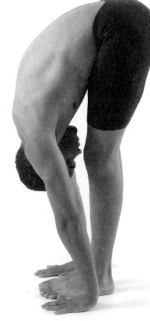

PHOTO 5.89

Goodman Photography

Forward-Stretch Pose (Uttāna Āsana) \oo-tah-nah-sa-na\

Preparation Stand in mountain pose [5.83]. Spread your feet hip-width apart, and keep them parallel.

The Exercise Inhale deeply. Exhale as you bend your knees slightly and drop your head forward. Continuing to exhale, bend your upper back forward and descend until you are hanging forward, your knees still slightly bent [5.88]. Breathe easily as you hang. Your fingers may touch the floor, or they may not. Either way, relax your arms and let them hang. Hold this for five to ten breaths. Then use an inhalation to help you rise back to standing, reversing the process by which you descended, so your head lifts up on top of your neck last.

To explore your stretch further, repeat the above pose, descending with an exhalation, and take three breaths in the pose. Then reach your fingertips toward the floor (or onto the floor) beside your feet while you hang your head and gently straighten your legs (they needn't be straightened all the way!). Finally, draw your head toward your legs [5.89]. Hold this pose for five to ten breaths, undulating slightly with your breath rhythm, and breathing into the stretch-feeling in your lower back.

To Finish Bend your knees and release your head. Then use an inhalation to rise, spine rounded, head hanging, until you at last lift your head onto the top of your spine. (This is called rolling up.) Stand in the mountain pose again. Sense your body for a few breaths.

Benefits This is one of the best and most versatile spinal flexion poses. Gravity aids the stretch, and it can be made safe for almost anybody by bending the knees and rounding the spine on the way down and on the way up. It stretches the hamstrings and the back. It inverts the torso, increasing blood circulation. And it increases your energy.

Cautions/Adjustments   The forward stretch is a natural position, one you use to reach your feet, tie your shoes, and so on, so it is quite safe. However, people who have a detached retina or glaucoma should avoid it. People who have disc problems should be careful and not force the pose, instead relaxing and letting gravity do the work.

The Deep Squat Pose (Utkat Āsana) \oot-kat-ah-sa-na\

Preparation   Stand in mountain pose [5.83], with your feet hip-width apart and parallel. Inhale. Then exhale into forward stretch pose [5.89].

The Exercise   Bend your knees enough to touch your fingertips to the floor in front of your toes. Lean forward to transfer some of your weight into your fingers and bend your knees,

descending into a deep squat, rising onto the balls of your feet. Position your knees in your armpits or just outside of your arms, keeping your feet parallel or nearly parallel. You may need to widen the distance between your feet. Relax your head forward and drape your arms out in front of you [5.90]. Let your heels rest on the floor if this is comfortable [5.91]. Sink downward, yielding to gravity. Breathe low in your lungs, so you feel the pressure of your inhalations all the way to the floor of your pelvis. Hold this pose for five to twenty breaths.

To Finish   Place your fingers or palms on the floor in front of your toes, lean forward, and press down hard as you straighten your legs into forward-stretch pose [5.89]. From there use an inhalation to roll up to mountain pose. Or you can continue from this pose into the warrior pose I, which follows.

Benefits   This pose is a natural position for our species. For millions of years our ancestors used this position for defecation and as a substitute for sitting on chairs. It imparts benefits so numerous that most anyone's health can be improved by performing this pose regularly. The deep squat pose tones your digestive organs, relieves constipation, stretches your calf muscles, soothes your lower back, opens your hip joints, and stimulates diaphragmatic breathing.

Cautions/Adjustments   If you feel pain in your ankles, place a folded blanket under your heels to support them. If you feel pain in your knees, support some of your weight with your hands or place a pillow between your ankles and your buttocks, thereby supporting your body with less bend in your knees. If you still feel pain in your ankles or knees, do not do this pose until you have worked with other āsanas for a while.

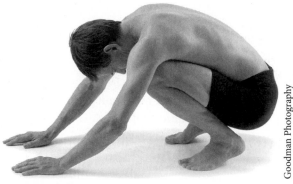

PHOTO 5.90

Goodman Photography

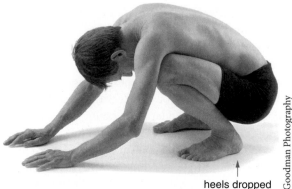

heels dropped

PHOTO 5.91

Goodman Photography

The Warrior Pose I, Variation (Vīrabhadra Āsana) \vee-ra-bha-drah-sa-na\

Preparation   Start in the forward stretch [5.89] or the deep squat [5.91], your hands beside your feet.

The Exercise   Step your left leg way back so that your right knee bends nearly ninety degrees and is over your ankle. Reach back through your left heel, flexing your ankle, and straighten your knee [5.92]. Hang your head for five to ten breaths, reaching forward with your bent right knee and back through your straightening left leg and through your heel.

You also can drop your left knee to the floor, if you need to [5.93]. Send your breaths into the stretching sensations in your left hip.

With an inhalation, raise your head and chest, straightening your arms and pressing through your fingertips into the floor. Reach into the floor through your feet and reach up through your spine and head. Square your shoulders and lower your pelvis toward the floor, bending your right knee more and tucking your tailbone under [5.94]. Gaze slightly upward. Your left knee may touch the floor, depending on your limberness. Hold this for three to eight breaths.

Repeat this on the other side, with your right leg stepping way back.

To Finish   Step forward into the forward stretch pose [5.89].

Benefits   The warrior pose I opens and stretches your hips, including a pair of important muscles for postural change, your iliopsoas. It strengthens your back muscles and relaxes your lower back.

Cautions/Adjustments   This pose can be modified by keeping your feet closer together than in the illustration and not bending your lead knee as much.

Downward-Facing Dog (Adho Mukha Svāna Āsana) \ad-ho moo-kha svah-nah-sa-na\

Preparation   Assume the forward stretch pose [5.89], with feet hip-width apart.

The Exercise   Walk your hands forward on the floor until you are in an upside-down "V" shape with your buttocks up. Drop your heels toward the floor, flexing your ankles and straightening your knees. Reach your sitting bones toward the ceiling. Press into the floor through your arms and hands, with fingers spread,

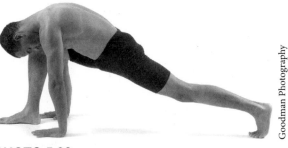

PHOTO 5.92

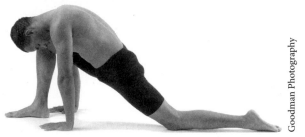

PHOTO 5.93

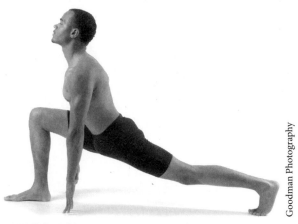

PHOTO 5.94

Goodman Photography

and reach your chest toward your feet, folding your body into more of a "V." Lengthen the back of your neck [5.95]. Rotate your shoulders outward, which drops them away from your ears slightly. Hold this pose for five to twelve deep breaths.

To Finish   Step one leg forward between your arms. Pause there. Then step the other leg forward to the forward stretch pose [5.89].

Benefits   This pose strengthens your arms, shoulders, and back. The inversion of your torso brings more blood circulation into your head. It stretches your hamstring and calf muscles.

Cautions/Adjustments   To make this pose more comfortable for your wrists, press through the whole of your palms instead of just the heel of your hand.

The Triangle Pose (Trikona Āsana) \tri-ko-nah-sa-na\

Preparation   Stand in mountain pose [5.83]. Step your feet about three to four and one-half feet apart, toes pointing forward. Raise your arms to shoulder height, palms down, and reach out through them, fingers reaching into the distance.

The Exercise   Turn out your right foot to aim it straight to the side, while turning your left foot to angle inward slightly. While reaching strongly through both arms, drop your right hand to your shin, to your right ankle, or to the floor outside of your foot, near your heel. Reach up vertically with your left arm and hand, your palm facing the way your chest faces. Look up toward your raised hand [5.96 and 5.97]. Hold the pose for three to twelve deep breaths, reaching out through your legs, your arms, and your spine.

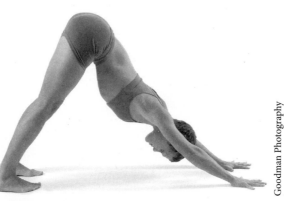

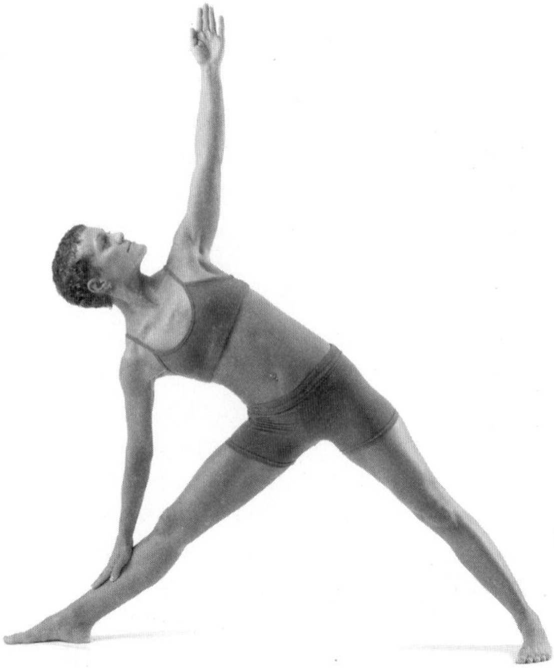

PHOTO 5.95

Goodman Photography

PHOTO 5.96

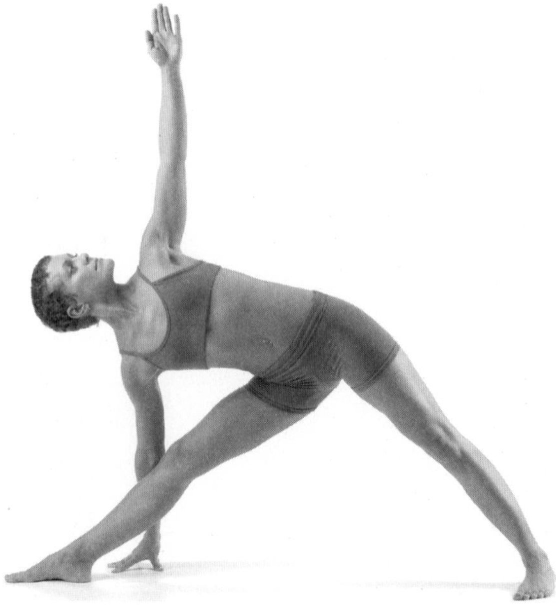

Goodman Photography

PHOTO 5.97

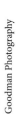

Goodman Photography

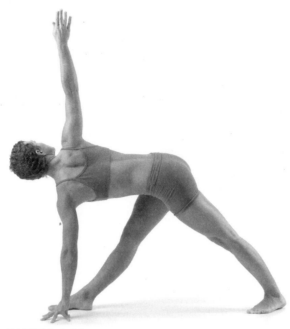

PHOTO 5.98

Goodman Photography

stop at your shin or ankle, clasp it. If your hand makes it to the floor, place your fingertips or palm on the floor. Reach your right arm away from your chest and raise it upward, toward vertical, palm aimed the way your chest aims.

Look up past your raised hand. Reach out through your limbs and through your spine [5.98]. Hold this pose and sense your muscles working, your limbs lengthening, for three to twelve breaths.

To Finish   Exhale completely. Then use the next inhalation to rise up to standing. Pivot your feet to parallel. Then turn out your left foot and turn in your right foot. Perform the pose on the other side, with your right hand reaching to your left leg or foot.

Benefits   This pose expands your diaphragmatic breath, reduces tension in your spine by twisting it, and strengthens your shoulders and neck.

Cautions/Adjustments   If your knee over which you are leaning hurts, bend it slightly and press down through your legs and feet into the floor, pulling up on your kneecaps by tightening your thigh muscles.

Warrior Pose II (Vīrabhadra Āsana) \vee-ra-bha-drah-sa-na\

Preparation   Stand in mountain pose [5.83]. Spread your feet wide apart so that your feet are under your wrists when you raise your arms to shoulder height, reaching out to the sides, palms down. Reach down from your pelvis through your legs into the floor. Reach up from your pelvis through your lower back, middle back, and neck. Reach out through your arms and fingertips, with your shoulders dropped.

The Exercise   Inhale deeply, turning your head to look to your right,

To Finish   With an inhalation, bend your right knee slightly and rise to standing erect. Now turn in your right foot, turn out your left foot, and repeat the pose on the other side.

Benefits   The pose strengthens your legs and back. It improves your hip range of motion. It enhances intercostal (mid-lung) breathing.

Cautions/Adjustments   If your front knee hurts, root both your feet into the floor and pull up on your kneecaps by tightening your thigh muscles. Or bend your front knee slightly.

Twisted Triangle Pose (Parivritta Trikona Āsana) \pa-ri-vrit-ta tri-kon ah-sa-na\

Preparation   Use the same preparation as for the triangle pose above.

The Exercise   Turn out your right foot to aim it straight to the side, while turning your left foot to angle inward slightly. While reaching strongly through both arms, twist and reach your left hand down to your right shin, ankle, or to the floor just inside of the ball of your foot. If you

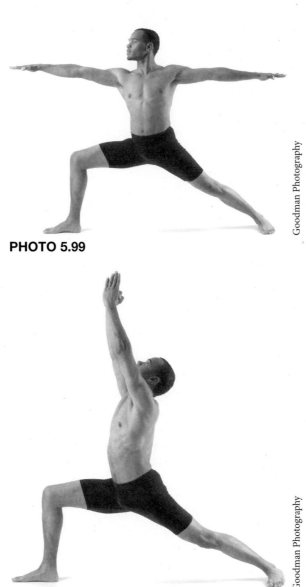

PHOTO 5.99

PHOTO 5.100

Goodman Photography

Goodman Photography

Warrior Pose I, Vīrabhadra Āsana

Preparation   Same as for warrior II, above.

The Exercise   Inhale deeply, turning your head to your right, turning out your right foot, and turning in your left foot. Breathe normally and rotate your torso, arms, and pelvis, so you face the direction your right toes point. You may need to pivot (turn in) your left foot more. Your pelvis now describes a line nearly perpendicular to the line made by your two feet, with your right hip slightly ahead of your left. With an inhalation, raise your arms sideways and overhead, bringing your palms together and hooking your thumbs. Exhale and bend your right knee. Breathe deeply and calmly as you lift your head and gaze upward, lifting your upper chest, lengthening your whole torso, and drawing your arms back as you continue to raise them [5.100]. Hold this pose for as long as you want to.

To Finish   With an exhalation, lower your straight arms to horizontal as you straighten your right leg. Then twist back to the front, rotating your feet.

Repeat the pose on the other side.

Benefits   Both warrior poses strengthen the core muscles in your back and abdomen. They stretch your calf muscles and elongate and strengthen your iliopsoas muscles in your hips. These warrior poses are among a very few that strengthen your iliopsoas muscles while they are in a fully lengthened position. This kind of strength aids you in many torso and leg movements, including walking and running. The warrior I also increases your shoulder joint strength and flexibility.

Cautions/Adjustments   When bending your knee, be careful to bend

simultaneously turning out your right foot so it aims directly away from you. Turn in your left foot slightly. Exhale and bend your right knee until your knee is over your ankle [5.99]. If you wish to intensify the pose, bend your right knee more, bringing your thigh to horizontal. Continue to reach throughout your body as you hold this pose for five to twelve breaths.

To Finish   Straighten your leg and turn your head and feet toward the front. Repeat the pose on the other side.

Benefits   See below for warrior I.

it straight over your foot, so if bent enough it would block your view of your foot. You direct this angle from your hip and by placing your foot so it aims the same way your knee is bending.

Intense Side-Stretch Pose (Pārsvōttana Āsana) \pahrs-voh-tan-ah-sa-na\

This is also called the intense chest stretch.

Preparation   Stand in mountain pose [5.83]. Spread your feet about two feet apart. Raise your arms to shoulder height, reaching out to the sides, palms down.

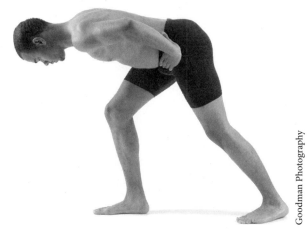

PHOTO 5.101

The Exercise   Turn out your right foot and turn in your left foot as for warrior pose, turning your upper body to your right to face your leg. (Adjust the angle of your left foot so your knee isn't twisting.) Inhale and bring your hands to your hips, then exhale and slightly bend your right knee, inclining forward, spine straight, until your back is horizontal or slightly higher [5.101]. Breathe normally and bend forward over your right leg, reaching down your leg, rounding your spine now, until you are as far forward as is comfortable. Straighten both legs, holding your leg or reaching your fingertips to the floor on either side of your foot. Press your left foot into the floor behind you, and lengthen your spine out of your pelvis, hanging your head toward your shin [5.102]. Hold this for three to eight breaths.

To Finish   Bend your right knee slightly and inhale as you rise to an upright stance, hands returning to your hips. Then turn toward the center, adjusting your feet to parallel. Perform the pose on the other side.

Benefits   This pose stretches your hamstring muscles and your back and strengthens your erector muscles.

Cautions/Adjustments   I recommend bending your lead knee as you incline forward and as you rise because this protects your knee. Straightening your knee in the transitions to this pose applies a hyper-extension force to it, stressing the ligaments. An alternative to bending your knee is to intensely contract your thigh muscles to stabilize your knee as you bend over it.

Side-Angle Pose (Pārsvakona Āsana) \pahr-sva-ko-nah-sa-na\

Preparation   Stand in a very wide stance, feet parallel, arms outstretched at shoulder height. Check that your feet are the same distance

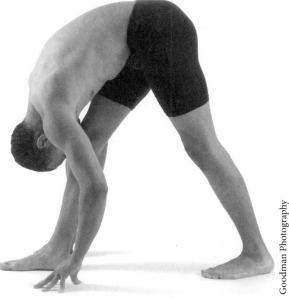

PHOTO 5.102

Goodman Photography

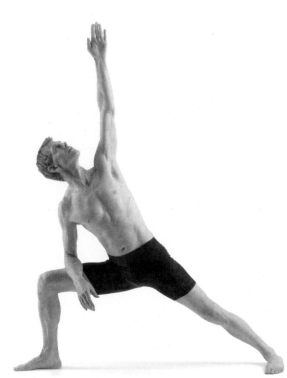

PHOTO 5.103

Goodman Photography

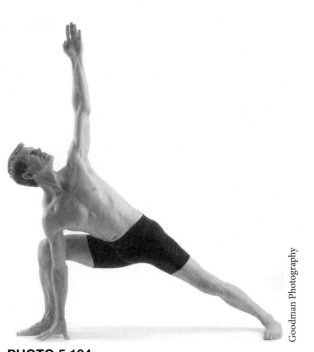

PHOTO 5.104

Goodman Photography

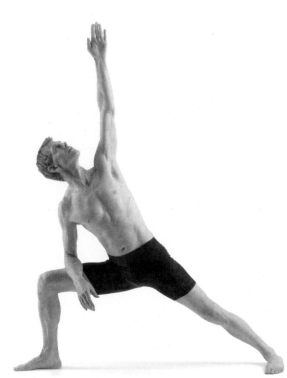

PHOTO 5.105

Goodman Photography

Exhale and bend your right knee until it is over your right ankle, pressing firmly into the floor through both feet. (This is warrior II.) Inhale again. Then exhale, reaching actively through your arms, inclining your torso and arms over your right leg until you can lean your forearm on your thigh, pressing down from your shoulder into your thigh, with your left arm now raised toward vertical, your chest opening to the front and your upper shoulder lifting and revolving back toward a position that is vertically over your lower one [5.103]. Keep the whole outside edge of your left foot down, adjusting the angle of your foot to allow this. Take a few deep breaths.

To continue further into the pose, reach your lower hand down to your ankle or to the floor on the inside of your right leg [5.104]. Hold this for a few breaths. Then incline your left arm overhead, to an incline equivalent to that of your side, or as close to that as is comfortable [5.105]. Keep opening your chest, drawing your left shoulder back. Gaze up, your neck staying in line with your spine. Continue reaching through your legs and feet, through your arms, and up through your spine, out the top of your head. Hold this pose for three to ten breaths.

apart as are the wrists of your outstretched arms.

The Exercise   Turn out your right foot ninety degrees, aiming it away from you, and turn in your left foot about forty-five degrees. Inhale.

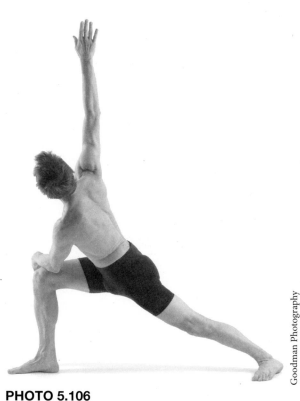

PHOTO 5.106

PHOTO 5.107

To Finish Raise your left arm to vertical. Inhale as you press down through both feet and rise to an erect-torso posture, right knee still bent, arms outstretched.

Use another inhalation to straighten your knee and turn your feet to parallel. Perform the pose on the other side.

Benefits This pose stretches and strengthens your pelvis and spine and opens your chest for deeper mid-lung and upper-lung breaths.

Cautions/Adjustments If your legs won't spread very far apart, proceed into the pose only as far as resting your forearm on your thigh.

Twisted Side-Angle Pose (Parivritta Pārsvakona Āsana) \pa-ri-vri-ta pahr-sva-ko-nah-sa-na\

Preparation Stand in a very wide stance, feet parallel, arms outstretched at shoulder height, as in the side-angle pose.

The Exercise Turn out your right foot ninety degrees, aiming it away from you, and turn in your left foot about forty-five degrees. Inhale. Exhale and bend your right knee until it is over your right ankle, pressing firmly into the floor through both feet. (This is warrior II.) Inhale again. Then exhale, reaching actively through your arms, *twisting your* torso to your right and bend toward your right leg until you can lean your left forearm on your thigh, pressing down from your shoulder into your thigh, with your right arm raised toward vertical, your chest opening, and your right shoulder lifting and revolving toward a position that is vertically over your lower one [5.106]. Keep the whole outside edge of your left foot down, adjusting the angle of your foot to allow this, reaching down through your legs from your pelvis. Take a few deep breaths.

To continue further into the pose, reach your left hand down to your ankle or to the floor on the inside of your right leg, reaching upward through your right arm and fingers [5.107]. Hold this pose for three to ten breaths.

Goodman Photography

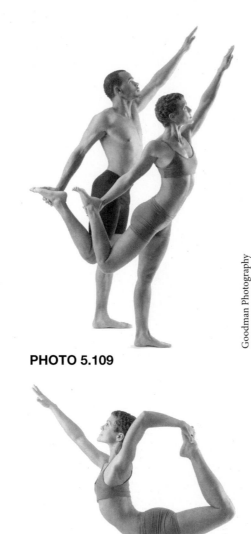

PHOTO 5.108

PHOTO 5.109

Goodman Photography

Goodman Photography

PHOTO 5.110

Goodman Photography

your abdominal oblique muscles, strengthens your thigh muscles, and stimulates diaphragmatic breathing.

Cautions/Adjustments   If your legs won't spread very far apart, proceed into the pose only as far as resting your forearm on your thigh. I recommend that you first learn the twisted side-angle pose from an experienced teacher.

Dancing Shiva Pose (Nātarāja Āsana) \nah-ta-rah-jah-sa-na\

Preparation   Stand in the mountain pose [5.83].

The Exercise   Balance on your left leg and bend your right leg to catch the top of your foot with your right hand behind you. Raise your left arm overhead [5.108]. Reach down through your standing leg and through your foot into the floor. Reach up through your spine and your lifted arm. Continue this as you engage your thigh muscles to straighten your right leg, but because you are holding it, your leg moves back, pulling your hand and foot back with it, and extending your spine. Your knee continues to point downward; your left arm and hand reach up and back. Tilt your body slightly forward to counterbalance your leg and arm behind you [5.109]. Hold the dancing Shiva pose with deep breaths, growing longer legs and arms, lifting up through your spine, and opening across the front of your chest. An advanced version of this pose is shown in Photo 5.110.

To Finish   Let your right knee bend, bringing your leg under you, returning to your preparatory pose [5.108]. Release to the mountain pose. Perform the pose on the other side.

Benefits   This pose improves your balance, strengthens your feet and ankles, extends your upper spine, and opens your chest and shoulders.

To Finish   Inhale as you press down through both feet and rise to an erect-torso posture, right knee still bent, arms outstretched. Use another inhalation to straighten your knee and turn your feet to parallel. Perform the pose on the other side.

Benefits   This pose strongly twists your spine, further releasing tension in your spine and chest. It strengthens

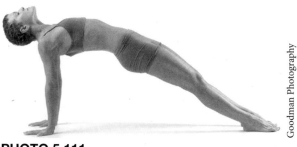

PHOTO 5.111

Goodman Photography

your legs, lengthening your neck, and tipping your head back slightly. Hold this for one to five breaths.

To Finish   Deeply inhale. Exhale as you sit down. Rest for a few breaths. Repeat the pose one or two more times. Then relax for a minute bent forward in the back stretch, paschim-ottana āsana, page 105 [5.77].

Benefits   This pose strengthens muscles in the backs of your legs, buttocks, torso, and shoulders, while stretching the front of your body. It prepares you for inversions. The front of body stretch especially strengthens muscles that help your shoulders to tolerate arm-supported facedown poses that are emphasized in the salutation to the sun, such as the four-footed staff pose [5.30], page 89). Anyone who frequently practices the salutation to the sun, or sequences of poses like it, should do this pose regularly.

Cautions/Adjustments   If you lack the strength to raise your pelvis, bend you knees in the pose. This pose re-quires substantial strength. Practice the locust pose group (starting on page 87) to develop this strength.

Cautions/Adjustments   If you have difficulty balancing on one leg, do this pose sideways to a wall.

Forward-Stretch Pose, Uttāna Āsana

This pose was taught earlier in the chapter, on page 109 [5.89].

Inversions

Note: A common caution given in Yoga classes regarding inversions, such as those that follow, is that menstruating women should not practice them. I address this concern in depth on page 149 in Chapter 7. I believe this decision is each woman's choice. There is no medical reason for a menstruating woman to avoid inversions.

Front-of-Body Stretch (Pūrvottāna Āsana) \poor-vo-than ah-sa-na\

This pose, which literally means east stretch, is an excellent preparatory pose for the inversions. It also pre-pares one's muscles for the salutation to the sun, which follows inversions.

Preparation   Sit on the floor, legs ex-tended, with your hands on the floor beside your hips.

The Exercise   Slide your hands back about eight inches, aiming your fin-gers behind you. Raise your pelvis up, pushing vigorously down through your hands, arms, and shoulders [5.111]. Point your toes, straightening

Shoulder Stand (Sarvānga Āsana) \sar-vahng ah-sa-na\

Preparation   Start in corpse pose, shava-āsana [5.5], but lying on a folded blanket (two inches thick), so that your upper back and shoulders are on the blanket and your neck and head rest on the floor.

The Exercise   Bring your knees up toward your chest and place your hands on your buttocks. While straightening your legs over your head, push your buttocks upward so your lower back lifts off the floor, your pelvis rising above you. Posi-tion your hands, fingers aimed toward your spine, on your back

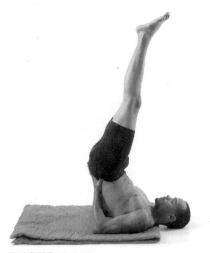

PHOTO 5.112

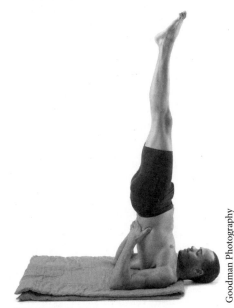

PHOTO 5.113

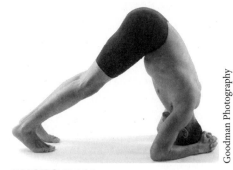

PHOTO 5.114

Goodman Photography

behind your hip bones, drawing your elbows closer together. Now raise your legs at an upward angle, while straightening them, until your feet are over your face. Support much of your weight with your arms [5.112]. Hold this pose for five to ten natural breaths.

To go further into the pose, walk your hands up your back as you raise your pelvis and legs higher, toward a vertical alignment [5.113]. Hold for thirty seconds to two minutes, with normal breathing.

To Finish   Reverse the order of movements to come down to the supine pose. Then immediately do a counter-pose, the fish pose [5.37, page 91], for three to five breaths.

Benefits   The shoulder stand stimulates circulation in your head and neck, as well as in your legs. It energizes you and calms your nervous system. The more vertical shoulder stand [5.113] compresses your chin into your throat and stimulates your thyroid gland.

Cautions/Adjustments   Be careful of your neck. I strongly recommend using a blanket as described when you do this pose, unless you are advanced at performing āsanas. Do not force yourself higher than feels comfortable in your neck and upper back. Avoid this pose if you have neck pain, cervical vertebrae problems, a detached retina, or glaucoma. Seek instruction from an experienced teacher before doing the more advanced shoulder stand, or if you experience neck discomfort in the easier version [5.112].

Head Stand (Shīrsha Āsana) \sheer-shah-sa-na\

Note: The head stand should be attempted only with the guidance of an expert instructor.

Preparation   Sit on your heels facing a wall about two to three feet in front of you. Lean forward and place your forearms on the floor, your fingers two inches from the wall. Interlace your fingers so the little-fingers edge of your hands is on the floor. Make two-thirds of an equilateral triangle with your forearms. Nestle your head into your palms with the top of your head on the floor (or place your head so that a spot about an inch in front of the top of your head presses into the floor).

The Exercise   Flex your feet and straighten your legs to nearly straight [5.114]. Walk your feet toward your head, raising your pelvis above your head and close to the wall. Bend one knee, bringing your heel close to your buttock, your thigh close to your chest. Attain a balance on the tripod of your head and your elbows. Hop your other foot up to join the first [5.115]. Lean into the wall behind you if you need to. (Always do this pose by a wall until you are an expert. A spotter is not a substitute for a wall.) Do not go any higher if you cannot balance in this position. Instead, keep practicing this preparatory pose.

To rise into the full head stand, unfold first your hips and then your knees to raise your legs straight above you. Hold your legs still and keep your feet touching [5.116]. Keep your abdominal muscles engaged to lengthen through your lower back and to draw the base of your rib cage toward your pubic bone. (You will need a teacher's guidance to achieve this. Adjusting your posture upside down is tricky.) Hold briefly.

To Finish   Bend your knees and hips slowly, maintaining balance, to lower your legs to the preparatory pose [5.115]. Lower one foot to the floor,

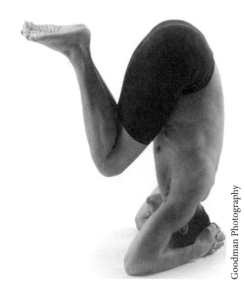

PHOTO 5.115

Goodman Photography

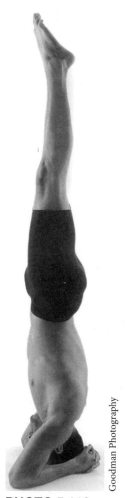

PHOTO 5.116

Goodman Photography

then the other. Walk your feet away and drop your knees down.

Go immediately into the counter-pose shown, the stretched child's pose (utthita bala āsana, pronounced oot-hi-ta ba-lah-sa-na) [5.117].

Reach through your arms as you breathe deeply against your upper spine for three to five breaths.

Benefits Called "the king of Yoga poses" in the Hatha Yoga literature, the head stand stimulates both your circulatory and your nervous systems in many ways, energizing you and increasing your awareness of sensations. It also strengthens your shoulders and neck, and improves your balance.

Cautions/Adjustments This is a difficult pose and must only be practiced with expert guidance. Those with eye problems, neck problems, or high blood pressure should not attempt it.

Tiger Breathing, Vyagrah Prānāyāma

This exercise was taught earlier in this chapter, on page 95 [5.50 and 5.51].

Corpse Pose, Shava-Āsana

Focus on your sensations of heaviness and your sensations of breathing for five to ten minutes.

Salutation to the Sun (Surya Namaskar) \soor-ya na-ma-skahr\

The Exercise Practice at least four rounds of the salutation to the sun

as shown [5.118]. Each round starts with position one, progresses through all the poses, and returns to position one. You may practice many more rounds if you wish.

To Finish End with the corpse pose, shava-āsana, sensing your heaviness and your breath for five minutes. Or go on to other poses. Standing twists complement the salutation series well.

Benefits The salutation to the sun strengthens your heart and lungs, stretches and strengthens many of your major muscle groups, and fully flexes and extends your spine. It is the most popular series of poses in the entire Yoga repertoire.

Cautions/Adjustments If you find the breathing instructions difficult to follow, do the āsana sequence with normal breathing. After familiarizing yourself with the poses and the sequence, try adding the breathing.

This series lacks twisting movements and side-bending movements, so it is best coupled with poses that achieve these ranges of motion.

Many people prefer to warm up before the salutation with easier poses.

If you practice the salutation often and for many repetitions, you should practice a counter-pose that helps prevent shoulder injuries. The front of body stretch, purvottana āsana, found on page 119 [5.111], strengthens muscles in your back, which balances the strengthening effect in your upper chest and the front of your shoulders.

Many variations on each pose exist, making this series accessible to anyone. Consult with your instructor to learn adjustments that are appropriate for you.

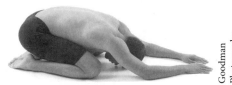

PHOTO 5.117

Goodman Photography

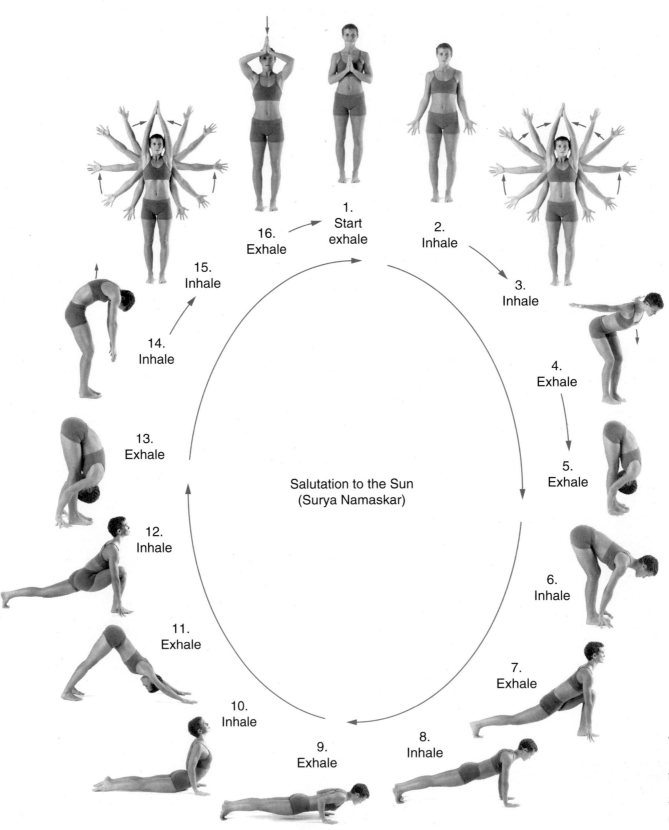

1.
Start
exhale

2.
Inhale

3.
Inhale

4.
Exhale

5.
Exhale

6.
Inhale

7.
Exhale

8.
Inhale

9.
Exhale

10.
Inhale

11.
Exhale

12.
Inhale

13.
Exhale

14.
Inhale

15.
Inhale

16.
Exhale

Salutation to the Sun
(Surya Namaskar)

Goodman Photography

PHOTO 5.118   Salutation to the sun

Relaxation and Meditation

Goodman Photography

The traditional goal of all Yoga practice is to clear your mind so you can see yourself and the world around you more clearly. Actually, the goal of Yoga is to completely clear your mind so you can see absolutely clearly. But on the way to ultimate clarity yogins notice degrees of change: the sky is blue-er, the sunshine is warm-er, a feeling of hunger is sharp-er. Every practice in every traditional Yoga system contributes in some way to this goal. But the practices that most directly clarify and intensify your hearing, seeing, or sensing are the practices of relaxation and meditation. We have seen that many other practices, such as postures and breath control, are traditionally used by yogins to condition their bodies and develop skills that they can then use in relaxation and meditation.

Relaxation and meditation are the final arena in which you clear your mind and experience your real self that has always been there, your *ātman*. We have seen that this mental clearing isn't easy because your mind is like a CD player stuck on play: your thoughts just keep coming, one thought triggering another, which reminds you of something that triggers another thought, and on and on (see Figure 6.1). Logically, you can't see past all this inner chatter unless

you can hit the stop button on your mental CD player. Your stop button is actually two buttons: one to disengage your attention from your thoughts and their scintillating content, and another to bring your attention into the present and focus it on one thing. The first button is relaxation; the second is concentration and meditation.

Relaxation

Every voluntary muscle in your body—that is, every muscle that you can consciously control—can be contracted or relaxed. Relaxed muscles use up less oxygen and glycogen (sugar) and discharge less carbon dioxide. Relaxed muscles also allow more blood to circulate and allow you to feel more sensation. Relaxation of muscles also leads to less mental activity.[1] In contrast, when you hold your muscles in a chronic contraction, your muscles use energy (glycogen), restrict blood flow, block subtle energy flow, cause an increase in mental activity, and tire you sooner. You can see that the ability to relax is essential to the

---

[1] Murphy, *The Future of the Body*, 405. Murphy discusses the research of Edmund Jacobson (1888–1983), who developed "Progressive Relaxation" in the early twentieth century. Murphy's book contains a list of thirty-two scientific studies conducted by Jacobson (pp. 624–625).

BOX 6.1

Yoga Experts Write About Relaxation

The state of Yoga is achieved by simultaneously striving and letting go.

—Patanjali, *Yoga Sutra* 1.12[2]

In [relaxation] the body is swept clean of the past, which is expressed in tensions and blockages in joints and muscles. Throughout the day and over the years, as the body accumulates the "fall-out" of emotional experiences and physical stress, it stores this "fall-out" in various parts of the body, such as the shoulders, the neck, the lumbar region and the hip joints. . . . Once the body has stored these negative energies, they become stuck to the point that most people are not even aware that they have a "problem." Before we can imprint a new type of awareness in the body, we have to relax the physical body, in whichever position it happens to be.

—Dona Holleman and Orit Sen-Gupta[3]

All techniques of Yoga aim to produce tranquility. Postures, breath controls, mind-stilling meditation, the bodily, mental, spiritual purifications—all have a relaxing influence that is widely acknowledged as probably Yoga's greatest advantage for Western man. For he lives at a pace unknown to his forefathers and his nervous system has to cope with a bombardment of stimuli that would have been intolerable to earlier generations.

—James Hewitt[4]

process of change that is central to Yoga. In this chapter we will explore general body relaxation, which works best if you practice it after you have performed Yoga āsanas for at least twenty minutes to half an hour. Relaxation of muscles works best if you have used your muscles repeatedly first, that is, after you are thoroughly warmed up. However, even if you haven't been exercising, the relaxation practices taught below will calm and recharge you any time you use them.

Benefits of Relaxation

Relaxation is the antidote to the stress of modern life. Like your need for sleep, you need downtime; you need islands of peace in your sea of urgent doing-going-seeking. All Yoga practices, including breathing and poses, provide you with a respite from your stimulating life. Yet relaxation practice takes you more deeply into peace, rest, ease, and pleasure than active practice can. Relaxation practice presses the stop button in your mind and slows down or suspends your emotional/mental agenda, your yearning, craving, "I"-building thoughts and emotions.

Regular relaxation practice also provides you with numerous physiological benefits, among them slower heart and respiratory rates, lower blood pressure, enhanced parasympathetic nervous system function (see "Benefits of Diaphragmatic Breath (Numbers 1, 2, and 3)," page 66, and Box 4.4, page 62, both in Chapter 4), improved immune system response, quicker reflexes, and more rapid recovery from stress.

---

[2] Desikachar, *The Heart of Yoga*, 113.

[3] Holleman and Sen-Gupta, *Dancing the Body of Light: The Future of Yoga*, 23.

[4] Hewitt, *The Complete Yoga Book*, 13.

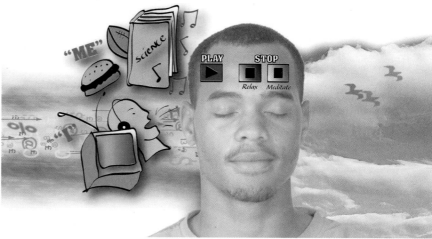

Photo: Leslie Goodman; Art: Kelly Burton

FIGURE 6.1   Your mind has two stop buttons. One is relaxation. The other is concentration and meditation.

Relaxation Exercises

Corpse Pose (Shava-Āsana) \sha-vah-sa-na\

These poses, which were taught in Chapter 4, can be done on a sticky mat (a plastic or rubber Yoga mat),

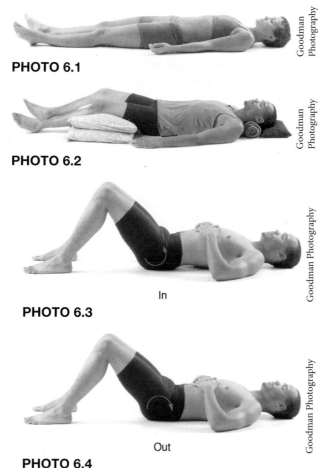

PHOTO 6.1

Goodman Photography

PHOTO 6.2

Goodman Photography

In

PHOTO 6.3

Goodman Photography

Out

PHOTO 6.4

Goodman Photography

on a thick blanket, on a rug, on a thin cotton-batting-style Yoga mat, on a lawn, or just about anywhere [6.1, 6.2]. You must remain warm throughout your practice in order to relax, so dress appropriately, or keep a blanket handy with which to cover yourself.

Relaxation Exercise #1: Pelvic Tilt in Modified Corpse Pose, Shava-Āsana

I teach this practice in Chapter 4, on breathing (page 58). It is both a breathing practice (*prānāyāma*) and a relaxation practice, and it is one of the best!

Benefits   In addition to the benefits described above for all Yoga relaxation exercises, the pelvic tilt with diaphragmatic breath [6.3, 6.4] rapidly engages your parasympathetic nervous system, whereas mid- and upper-chest breathing engage your sympathetic nervous system. (See "Benefits of Diaphragmatic Breath (Numbers 1, 2, and 3)," page 56.) This means that diaphragmatic breath lowers your blood pressure, increases digestion, awakens your internal sensations, makes you aware of your emotions, and enables your mind to work more creatively. All these effects accompany the functioning of your parasympathetic nervous system, which you use when you are feeling safe, unworried, and comfortable.

Relaxation Exercise #2, Breath Watching (Prāna Jnāna Kriyā) \prah-na nyah-na kree-yah\

This translates to "vital-energy wisdom exercise."

Preparation   Lie in the corpse pose or modified corpse pose [6.1, 6.2]. Relax your whole body, feeling the places where you press into the floor. Surrender your weight to the floor. Continue this weight-focus for two minutes.

The Exercise   Switch your focus to your breathing sensations, feeling your breath coming in, and feeling it going out. Don't interfere with your natural breathing or try to control it in any way. Just notice it as it is.

Notice the many sensations that arise as you breathe: the movement of air in your nostrils, cool coming in, warm going out; the flow of air down your throat; and the movements of your chest, belly, sides, and back. As you notice all this, let your breath do whatever it wants. Let it come in deeply at times. Let it stop briefly if it wants. Let it be erratic or regular.

Notice how different your inhalations feel from your exhalations: Your inhalations involve effort and contractions of muscles such as your diaphragm and your between-the-ribs muscles (intercostals), while your exhalations involve relaxation, a letting go in all those muscles.

Focus into the exhalation phase of each breath, which is the relaxation phase. See if you can let go even more deeply than you ordinarily do with each of your exhalations.

Notice how your breathing feels at the end of your inhalation, just before you start to exhale. Does your breath pause? Does it slow down, like a ball thrown skyward that is just reaching the top of its arc? Notice how your breathing feels at the end of your exhalation. Does your breath stop for an instant before you start to inhale again? If your breath stops briefly here, pay close attention to how that moment of pause feels.

Feel free to tour your breathing sensations, moving your awareness to another sensation or to another area of your body whenever you want.

Continue this breath exploration for ten to fifteen minutes. Whenever you notice that your mind has become occupied with thoughts, and is no longer focused on breathing sensations, gently bring it back to your body and your sensations of breathing. It is OK if this mental retrieval happens many times. In this exercise, dealing compassionately with your wandering mind is as important as focusing on your sensations.

To Finish   Sense your whole body. Begin moving your fingers and toes, feeling them. Let the movement spread to your arms and legs, feeling them. Move any way that your limbs want to, without thinking about it or directing them.

Now move any way that your body feels like moving, breathing spontaneously, for a minute or two. Then roll onto your side in order to rise to a sitting position.

Cautions/Adjustments   If lying on your back in the corpse pose becomes uncomfortable within ten minutes, use props as described in cautions/adjustments for the corpse pose in Chapter 5 (page 81).

Benefits   This relaxation calms you rapidly and attunes you to your inner energy, called *prāna*. With practice, this energy will become increasingly more apparent to you. As this happens, your emotions will become more apparent, too.

BOX 6.2

Science Investigates Relaxation

The practice taught in Exercise 3 bears some resemblance to another practice, called "Progressive Relaxation," developed by Edmund Jacobson (1888–1983), which was extensively researched between 1911 and 1974.[5] Vital point relaxation predates his work and is mentioned in three Upanishads—Shandilya-Upanishad (1.8.1f.), Kshurika-Upanishad (14), and Darshana-Upanishad (7.1-2).[6] Today, relaxation practices such as vital point relaxation are widely taught in Yoga classes. We know much more about their possible effects because of Jacobson's research, because even though his techniques were not identical to the ones mentioned in the Upanishads, they are similar enough for us to surmise that the positive benefits shown in scientific research for Progressive Relaxation also apply to those practicing Yoga relaxation. More recent research into the effects of specific Yoga relaxation practices and into non-Yoga relaxation techniques have added to our understanding. The evidence suggests that regular relaxation practice imparts numerous preventative and healing benefits.[7]

Relaxation Exercise #3, Vital Point Relaxation (Marman Kriya) \mar-man kree-ya\

This exercise is also called *yoga nidrā* (pronounced yo-ga nid-rah′), meaning yoga sleep.

Preparation Lie in the corpse pose or modified corpse pose. Sense your breathing, as you did in breath watching above, for a few minutes.

The Exercise Focus on your big toes, feeling them and telling them to let go. Say to your big toes, "Let go" or "Relax." Stay with your toes for about thirty seconds.

Focus on your feet, feeling them and telling them to let go or relax, for about thirty seconds. Notice the pressure against the floor in the backs of your heels. Feel both your skin and the insides of your feet.

Focus on your ankles, feeling them and telling them to let go or relax. Feel both the insides and the surfaces of your ankles.

Continue in the same way throughout your body in these stages: calves, shins, knees, thighs, anus, genitals, belly and lower back, heart and middle back, hand and wrist, elbow and upper arm, shoulders, neck and throat, the root of your tongue, back of your palate, the root of your nose, the space between your eyebrows, forehead and temples, top of your head [6.5]. This whole process takes from ten to fifteen minutes.

To Finish Sense your whole body at once. As you are sensing, begin moving your arms and legs spontaneously, stretching or wiggling any way your body wants. Return to sitting when you feel ready to.

Benefits Vital point relaxation produces all the benefits of Yoga relaxation that I listed above (page 125).

Cautions/Adjustments If you need to increase your comfort in the corpse pose, use props as described in cautions/adjustments for the corpse pose in Chapter 5 (page 81).

---

[5] Murphy, *The Future of the Body*, 624–625.

[6] The first two Upanishads are cited in Feuerstein, *The Shambhala Encyclopedia of Yoga*, 183; the third is cited in Johari, *Chakras*, 105.

[7] Murphy, *The Future of the Body*, 399–405.

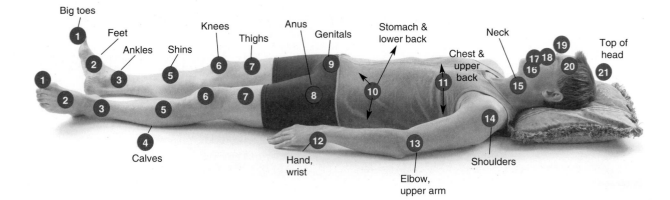

Big toes · Feet · Knees · Thighs · Anus · Genitals · Stomach & lower back · Neck · Top of head · Ankles · Shins · Chest & upper back · Calves · Hand, wrist · Elbow, upper arm · Shoulders

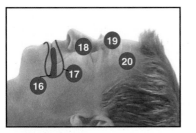

16. Root of tongue
17. Back of your palate
18. Foot of nose
19. Between eyebrows
20. Forehead & temples

PHOTO 6.5

Relaxation Exercise #4, Tense and Release Relaxation (Dridha Kriya) \dri-dha kree-ya\

This literally means "firming action."

Preparation   Lie in the corpse pose or modified corpse pose. Relax your whole body, feeling the places where you press into the floor and relaxing there. Surrender your weight to the floor. Take three easy deep breaths.

The Exercise   Part 1. Reach your arms overhead. As you inhale deeply, stretch up through your arms and down through your feet, engaging your whole body in the stretch, elongating your entire body. As you complete your inhalation, keep stretching. Hold your breath in briefly.

Suddenly let your breath rush out in a whoosh. At the same time suddenly relax and go limp—arms, legs, everything. Sense your relaxed body for a moment, your breath moving automatically.

Reach overhead again and repeat the stretching inhalation, hold . . . and go limp. Repeat once more, three times total.

Part 2. With your arms overhead, in the same way as before, inhale and stretch both up and down, but as you do roll onto your *left* side. Hold your breath and hold the stretch, intensifying it, remaining on your side.

Suddenly go limp as you let your breath rush out with a whoosh, flopping onto your back. Roll from your side onto your back as limply as you can.

Repeat this while rolling onto your *right* side. Do six of these side stretches total, three on each side.

To Finish   Straighten your body out and bring your arms down along your sides, so you are again lying in the corpse pose. Rest here for five minutes, doing nothing. When you feel ready to get up, roll onto your side or stomach first, then rise to sitting from there.

BOX **6.3**

Yoga Experts Write About Meditation

Pleasure and love are the way; they are not the goal. It is necessary to go beyond them to reach it. Cerebral thought, on the other hand, is the obstacle, that centripetal organ which makes each of us the center of the world and prevents us from giving ourselves up and finally dissolving in the perception of the beauty of forms, then cosmic harmony, and finally the creative thought.

—Alaine Daniélou[8]

Consciously or unconsciously we are all seeking the peace of mind that meditation brings. All of us have our own ways of finding this peace, our own meditative habits—from the old lady who sits knitting by the fire to the boatman whiling away a summer's afternoon by the river, oblivious to the passing of time. For when our attention is fully engaged, the mind becomes silent; when we succeed in restricting our thoughts to one object the incessant internal chattering stops. Indeed the contentment we feel when our minds are absorbed often comes less from the activity itself than from the fact that in concentrating our worries or problems are forgotten.

—Lucy Lidell[9]

Cautions/Adjustments   Do not hold your breath if you have elevated blood pressure. Simply do the practice without the holding-in part.

Benefits   This relaxation is useful when you are tired and unable to concentrate. It increases your energy while at the same time relaxing you. The loose flopping onto your back from a side-lying position is excellent for your spine.

Meditation

Note: The English word *meditation* applies to both Yoga concentration, *dhāraṇā* (pronounced dha-ra-nah), and Yoga meditation, *dhyāna* (pronounced dhy-ah-na). When the word *meditation* is used in a technical sense to discuss Yoga practices or states attained through Yoga practice, it usually refers to dhyāna. Most everywhere else it means both dhāraṇā and dhyāna. I use the word *meditation* both ways below.

Benefits of Meditation

Meditation has existed in human societies since the beginning of recorded history. Instructions in its methods, and the motivation to practice it, have been passed from person to person, generation to generation for at least five thousand years. Meditation's benefits were apparently substantial for this to have happened. I have described these benefits, as viewed through the Yoga tradition, throughout this book. The central one is that meditation, when practiced consistently over many years, alters one's perceptions and one's sense of self. The meditator's former sense of being a separate thing, different from and cut off from everything and everyone around her, is replaced with a sense of similarity with and a union with everything around her. Students of mine have described this as feeling like coming home.

---

[8] Daniélou, *Yoga: Mastering the Secrets of Matter and the Universe,* 8.

[9] Lidell, *The Shivananda Companion to Yoga,* 89.

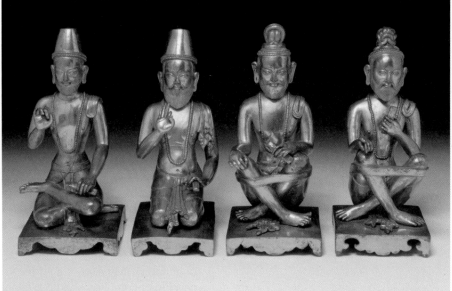

V&A Images, London/Art Resource, NY

PHOTO 6.6   A group of yogins in meditation postures. Nepal, 18th century.

In the early nineteenth century scientists became interested in the phenomenal abilities of religious adepts. Tales of remarkable feats led researchers to attempt to determine if such tales were real. The sorts of religious adepts who were investigated included Catholic saints whose hands and feet bled, a Chuckchee shaman performing primitive surgery that left no scars, and a yogin surviving six weeks of burial.[10] Many of these feats appeared to be real, although skeptics have long claimed that sleight of hand or some kind of trickery offer a more plausible explanation for supposedly supernormal abilities.

Less flashy meditation practices came under the scientist's microscope starting in the 1930s[11] and especially after 1970, during which time over 1,300 studies have been published in journals, books, or graduate theses—and those are just the studies in English![12] (There have been many more studies conducted on meditation than on relaxation.) An interesting picture has emerged of meditation's effects, which vary; some

effects appear consistently, whereas other effects have not been consistent. One problem with meditation research has been that the subjects used in the studies have mostly been novices. As Michael Murphy writes in *The Future of the Body*:

> The results of meditation research are accumulating now in the manner of scientific knowledge generally, forming a publicly accessible body of empirical data that can serve generations to come. Unfortunately, however, these data are derived mainly from meditation beginners, and taken as a whole do not reflect the richness of experience described in traditional contemplative teachings. They are also limited by the conventional scientific insistence that results be repeatable. Certain important experiences occur only rarely in meditation, and a science that disregards them loses much of its empirical results. For these reasons, contemporary research does not illumine the full range of experience described in the contemplative scriptures and the oral traditions from which they come.[13]

---

[10] Murphy, *The Future of the Body*, 527.

[11] Ibid.

[12] Ibid., 538.

[13] Ibid., 539.

In spite of these limitations, research results have largely shown benefits to meditation. These health benefits, along with meditators' anecdotal reports, have inspired many people to add fifteen minutes to an hour of meditation to their daily lives. These benefits overlap substantially with the benefits of relaxation, listed above, and also extend beyond them. Meditation's benefits, supported by research, include the following:[14]

Lowered resting heart rate

Reduced blood pressure in people who are normal or mildly hypertensive (not in people with acute hypertension)

Synchronization of brain wave activity between the right and left hemispheres and the anterior and posterior parts of the brain

Reduced oxygen consumption, carbon dioxide elimination, and respiration rate, suggesting a lowered need for energy and the oxygen to metabolize it

Reduced muscle tension and blood lactate associated with reduced anxiety

Reductions in stress symptoms such as increased skin resistance and salivary changes

Rapid recovery from stress as indicated by skin conductance, heart-rate, self-report, and fewer activations of the flight-or-fight response

Reduction in chronic pain

Enhanced perception, such as visual sensitivity and auditory acuity

Improved reaction time

Increased ability to concentrate

Relief from addictions

Increased energy

Increased dream recall

Decrease in migraine headaches

Decrease in premenstrual syndrome symptoms

Reductions in insomnia

Increased immune system function

Decreased panic attacks

Guidelines for Meditation

The essential guideline for success in meditation is simple: sit, notice, keep sitting. But sitting still for ten or fifteen minutes isn't so simple. Here are some situations you may confront, and some helpful guidelines for each situation.

You may find that your thoughts seem to fill your awareness when you sit down to meditate, even more than they do at other times. That's OK. Keep sitting and focusing. Let your thoughts be there.

The thoughts that appear in your mind may seem urgent. You may think, "I have to write my mother and thank her for that gift RIGHT NOW!!!" Or, you may think, "I HAVE TO check that the cat has water in her dish right now." You can do it later. You won't forget. Keep sitting. If you yield to your mind at such moments and get up to do its bidding, you will find it harder to meditate when you sit back down. Keep sitting. Remember that Yoga practice develops in a person a capacity to tolerate strong feelings. (See "Feeling Emotions" in Chapter 5, page 76.)

If you are often critical of yourself, you may think, "I'm just not very good at meditation. Maybe others can do it, but I guess it's not for me." Everyone thinks this at first. It isn't true. Anybody can meditate. Keep going. Be patient.

Everyone hates to be bored. When you are bored you may feel

---

[14] Ibid., 603–610; Khalsa and Stauth, *Meditation as Medicine*, 42–46.

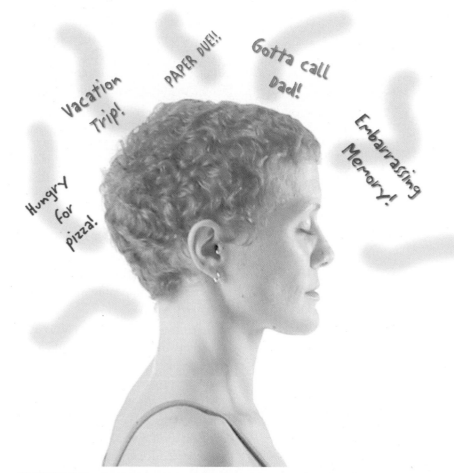

PHOTO 6.7   Some people find that their thoughts seem to become loud and insistent when they sit down to meditate. That's OK. Let your thoughts be there.

frustration, impatience, irritation, or itches that appear all over your body. You may feel uncomfortable sensations related to your sitting pose that make you want to squirm, or you may feel impulses to do something impish (especially if you are meditating with other people). Boredom is your friend. Don't do any of the above things. Don't scratch (OK, maybe once or twice), don't squirm, and don't make rude noises. Keep sitting.

Many people think critical thoughts about their teacher or the meditation instructions themselves. Don't dwell on them. Come back to your focus and let them be. This is not a time to figure anything out.

You may find yourself reviewing incidents when someone hurt you, or incidents when you did something you regretted. When you notice that you are thinking such things, come back to your focus and keep sitting.

Cautions

If you are taking prescription medications for mood disorders, ask your doctor before starting a meditation practice.

Don't practice when under the influence of recreational drugs.

If you have medical conditions such as epilepsy or depression, consult a physician before beginning a meditation practice.

Do not meditate for more than one hour per day unless instructed to do so by an expert instructor

Preparation for Meditation

Prepare the Space and Choose a Time

Prepare an area in your house or your room for your meditation practice. It should be clean and unstuffy, and should smell good. You can also meditate outdoors in a place where you won't be disturbed and where you feel completely safe. Being suddenly interrupted in the middle of meditation is jarring to your nervous system. If you are indoors, choose a time for your meditation when you won't be disturbed, or tell your housemates what you are doing and ask not to be interrupted until you are done. Wait at least one and one half hours after a meal to begin your practice.

Prepare Your Seat

If indoors, elevate your buttocks by sitting on a folded-up blanket or pillows, so that your knees are at the level of you hips or lower [6.8]. Meditation cushions are available in many larger bookstores and in all metaphysical bookstores as well as online. If you meditate outdoors, you may be more comfortable sitting on a slight slope, so your legs rest on the ground at a lower level than your buttocks.

Choose a Sitting Pose, Āsana

The traditional meditation poses are ones in which your legs are crossed, your back is erect, and you are not leaning against anything, as shown in 6.8 and 6.9. But this kind of pose is only appropriate for meditation if you can sit this way comfortably for the length of time you have allotted. If discomfort in the pose makes you stop meditating, you are in the wrong pose. Alternatives to traditional poses include sitting cross-legged against a wall [6.10] or in a chair with back support [6.11], or sitting in a chair, your feet on the floor, without leaning back [6.12].

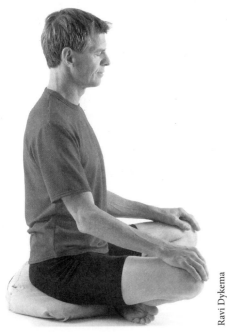

PHOTO 6.8

Ravi Dykema

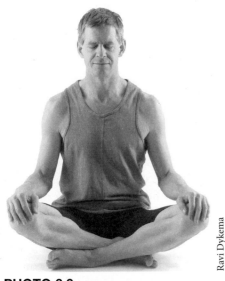

PHOTO 6.9

Ravi Dykema

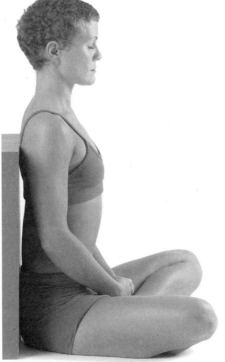

PHOTO 6.10

Goodman Photography

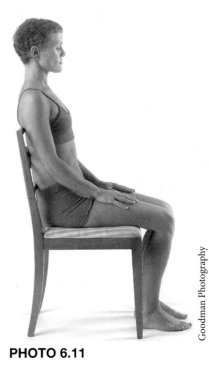

PHOTO 6.11

Goodman Photography

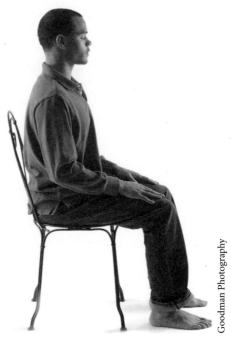

PHOTO 6.12

Goodman Photography

A List of the Six Meditation Practices Taught Elsewhere in This Book

In Chapter 1 I teach four meditation practices, one for each of these four branches of Yoga: Bhakti Yoga (p. 8), Mantra Yoga (p. 8), Jnana Yoga (p. 10), and Raja Yoga (p. 11). In Chapter 3 I teach a Hatha Yoga concentration practice called "vital energy focus," prāṇa dhāraṇā (p. 40). In Chapter 4 I teach a breath practice that, if done in a meditative sitting pose such as those illustrated above, is a meditation practice. It is called "Natural Breath Awareness: The Autonomic Breath" (p. 55).

Practices of Meditations

After trying each of these three practices, as well as the six referred to in Box 6.4, for a day or two, choose the meditation practice that you like the most and practice it every day, or every other day, at about the same time each day. Commit to two weeks of this practice before you consider changing your practice to a different one, or before you decide to give it up. Meditation's benefits aren't instant. You may experience wonderful results from your practice even if the first few weeks of it were difficult.

Start out meditating for fifteen minutes each time. (This will take you about twenty minutes because of the time it takes to get situated and the time it takes to return to activity.) After a week, extend the time to twenty or thirty minutes of meditation.

Meditation #1, Breathing with "Om" Meditation

Preparation   Sit in your favorite meditation pose, having prepared your space. Close your eyes and relax as much as you can without slouching or sagging. Keep your head up. Don't tip it forward as if you were looking down.

To Begin   Turn your attention to your body and your sensations. Survey your whole body slowly, part by part, in no particular order, noticing your sensations in each part. Relax a little more as you do this. Take about three minutes for this inventory of your sensations.

The Concentration   Place your attention on your breathing, feeling the sensations of your breathing in your nostrils, in your throat, in your chest, and in your belly and back. Allow your breath to be automatic for about a minute, while you focus on your sensations of breathing. Throughout this practice, keep breathing through your nostrils.

Begin controlling your breath. (It will be helpful if you have completed all the exercises given in Chapter 4, but not essential.) Inhale slowly as you count, "one, two, three, four." Then exhale slowly as you count, "one, two, three, four." Continue counting four in, four out, with your breaths. A count of about one per second is fine. Discover your own rhythm. It should feel easy, unhurried. Relax your throat, so your breath doesn't make a sound in it. If, after a few counted breaths, you are still feeling uncomfortable, try

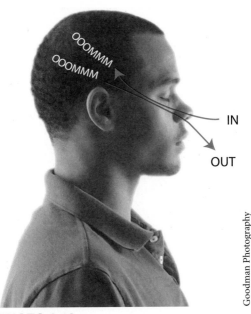

PHOTO 6.13

Goodman Photography

and counting your breaths. Whenever you find that you aren't counting, or thinking the sound om, or sensing your breathing, just bring your attention to these points again. It is OK for your mind to wander many times. This is natural. Just keep bringing your attention back to the practice.

To Finish   Let your breathing become automatic, stopping the counting and thinking om. Sense your body for a minute or so: your buttocks pressing into the seat, the sensations in your back, the sensations in your arms and head. Then stretch, rub your face, whatever you spontaneously feel like doing before getting up.

Meditation #2, The "I Am Well" Meditation, with the So Ham Mantra

So ham (pronounced so-hum) means "I am that," with "that" referring to the ultimate reality, your true self, your highest self, or the beingness of everything.

Preparation   Sit in your favorite meditation pose, having prepared your space. Close your eyes and relax as much as you can without slouching or sagging. Keep your head centered and level.

To Begin   Turn your attention to your body and your sensations. Survey your whole body slowly, part by part, in no particular order, noticing your sensations in each part. Relax a little more as you do this. Take about three minutes for this inventory of your sensations.

The Concentration   Place your attention on your breathing, feeling the sensations of your breathing in your nostrils, in your throat, in your chest, and in your belly and back. Allow your breath to be automatic while you focus on your sensations of breathing.

speeding up your breathing slightly by counting three in, three out. Experiment and find a depth and pace that feels easy and natural to you. If after about five breaths you still feel uncomfortable, relax your breath completely and return to normal uncontrolled breathing. When you are ready to try controlling your breath again, dispense with counting entirely and just breathe in and out a little more slowly and a little more deeply than you do ordinarily.

After you become accustomed to controlling your breath as just described, add a sound. Think "oooooommmmm" (sounds like "h**ome**") as you inhale, for the whole four counts (or three counts). Then think "oooooommmmmm" as you exhale, for the whole count [6.13]. Continue thinking om with each of your inhalations and exhalations. Focus on the sound while you also focus on your sensations of breathing. Continue this practice for the whole time you have intended to meditate.

If you find this difficult, just practice om on the exhalation.

Many thoughts will intrude, some demanding your full attention. Let them come and go. Keep thinking om

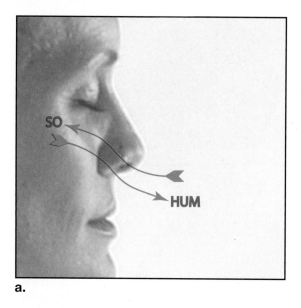

a.

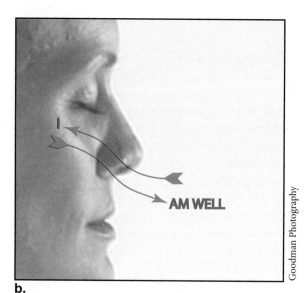

b.
FIGURE 6.2

Goodman Photography

While you inhale, think "I." When you exhale, think "am well" (Figure 6.2b). Continue this sound, along with your breath, for the duration of your meditation.

Many thoughts will intrude, some demanding your full attention. Let them come and go. Keep thinking "so ham" or "I am well." Whenever you find that you aren't thinking the sound, or aren't sensing your breathing, just bring your attention to these points again. It is OK for your mind to wander many times. This is natural. Just keep bringing your attention back to the practice.

To Finish   Stop thinking the sound. Return to normal breathing. Sense your body for a minute or so, and then stretch, rub your face, or do whatever you spontaneously feel like doing before getting up.

Meditation #3, Third Chakra Meditation (Manipūra Chakra Dhāranā) \mu-ni-poo-ra chah-krah dha-ra-nah\

Tantra Yoga and Hatha Yoga both contain many concentration practices that direct the yogin's attention within his or her body, to a single point. This is one of those practices. For more information on *chakras*, consult Chapter 3, "The Anatomy of Awakening: *Kundalinī* and *Chakras*," page 42.

Preparation   Sit in your favorite meditation pose, having prepared your space. Close your eyes and relax as much as you can without slouching or sagging. Keep your head centered and level.

To Begin   Turn your attention to your body and sensations: Survey your whole body slowly, part by part, in no particular order, noticing your sensations in each part. Relax a little more as you do this. Take about three minutes for this inventory of your sensations.

Throughout this practice, breathe automatically through your nostrils. Let your breath do whatever it wants to do, such as yawn, or sigh, or move more quickly or slowly. Don't control it; just notice.

While you continue to feel your breathing, think "so," as in "*so*ul," during your in breath; and think "ham," as in "hum," during your out breath (Figure 6.2a). Continue this focus on breath and sound for the whole meditation.

Or, you may change the sound after awhile to a loose English translation of so ham, which is "I am well."

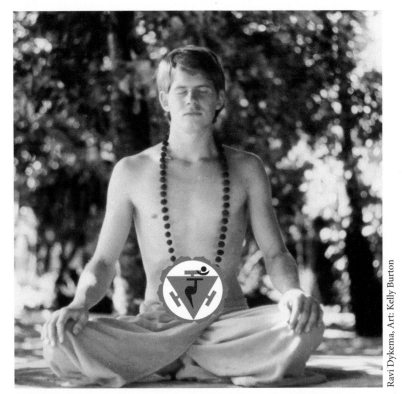

PHOTO 6.14 In Tantra Yoga, the third chakra is depicted in a graphic form. The chakra shown, manipūra chakra, is near the solar plexus.

Ravi Dykema, Art: Kelly Burton

The Concentration Place your attention on your breathing, feeling the sensations of your breathing in your nostrils, your throat, your chest, and your belly and back. Allow your breath to be automatic while you focus on your sensations of breathing. Throughout this practice, keep breathing automatically through your nostrils. Let your breath do whatever it wants to do naturally, such as yawn, or sigh, or move more quickly or slowly. Don't control it; just notice.

After a few minutes of watching your breath, bring your focus to your navel. Then sense under your navel, inside your belly, into a place that feels like your middle, your gut-sense place, your center of gravity. This is easy to find. Just settle your awareness wherever it naturally goes. If it moves after a while, that is OK, too. This spot inside you may be slightly higher or lower than your navel. If you can't

find the spot, focus five inches behind your navel. Don't worry about being exact.

Hold your attention at this point, gently settling your awareness in your belly as a butterfly would settle on a flower. Relax, breathe naturally, and sense your belly spot. Continue this for the duration of your meditation.

Let your thoughts come and go. Keep focusing in your belly. Whenever you find that you aren't sensing your belly spot, just bring your attention to it again. It is OK for your attention to wander off into thoughts many times. This is natural. Just keep bringing your attention back to the practice, over and over.

To Finish Sit quietly. Sense your whole body for a few minutes, noticing your feelings in your legs, your arms, your chest, and your head. Then stretch, rub your face, wiggle—whatever you spontaneously feel like doing. After a minute or so of this, get up.

Using Meditation Practices Already Presented in This Book

You can also use any of the practices I have already given (listed above in box) in a daily practice. Simply adjust them as follows: prepare your meditation space, your seat, and choose a pose as described above.

Try all the practices given, doing each one for one to two days. Do your meditation for at least fifteen minutes, but no more than thirty minutes. (The previously given meditation instructions suggest a shorter time because they were initially intended to be done while you were reading this book. To make them even more effective, do them as suggested here, for fifteen to thirty minutes.) Keep a watch or clock handy with which to time yourself.

Integrating Meditation into Your Life

Choose one meditation technique from among the ones you have tried and practice it daily for one month. Then try skipping a week. Notice how you feel, how you react to stressful situations, and how your studies go. If you are like many others, you will find that you have been enjoying benefits from meditation that developed gradually, which you didn't notice until they were gone. This may inspire you to meditate most days for many years, or for the rest of your life. If this happens, I think you will see even more clearly how your activities, your food choices, your sleep cycles, your Yoga āsana classes—how all these affect your meditation and your health. With this new awareness, you may be able to achieve more contentment, more compassion for others, more success in your endeavors, and more peace. This is the potential of Yoga.

Yoga for Special Needs

Goodman Photography

Yoga Classes Are for Everybody

While it may seem to you that only healthy or already-athletic people are candidates for Yoga classes, this is not true. Yoga's diverse methods can accommodate nearly anyone who wants to become healthier or who wants to see themselves and the world more clearly.

Most modern Yoga teacher trainings contain elements of Yoga therapy (more on Yoga therapy below) so that most Yoga teachers can accommodate a variety of body types and levels of fitness among their students.

I have worked as a Yoga therapist with elderly people with terminal illnesses who required supplemental oxygen; I have worked with people who have spinal cord injuries and must use a wheelchair; and I have worked with people who live with chronic pain. People in all three groups (and others) have benefited from Yoga practice. The system of Yoga is versatile. Its many movement, breath, and concentration practices can be adapted to people in just about any situation.

This chapter will help you adapt the Yoga system taught in this book, and the Yoga system taught in the classes you are taking, to your needs, whether you are unfit, pregnant, overweight, recovering from an injury, or have some other kind of strength or movement restriction.

You Can Do It

The key principal for you is, "You can do it." You can listen to your body, notice your sensations, modify ordinary Yoga exercises, and create a practice that gives you wonderful results.

This chapter describes how you can adapt the Yoga teachings to your body, and thereby gain pain relief, comfort, confidence, and improvements in your health. We'll cover how to adapt Yoga to your body:

If you are overweight or out of shape

If you are experiencing chronic pain

If you are experiencing back pain

If you are pregnant

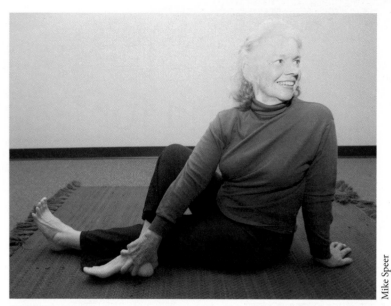

Mike Speer

PHOTO 7.1   Anyone can do Yoga poses.

Note: People who are disabled, who have severe chronic pain, or who have serious illnesses should seek the help of a thoroughly trained Yoga therapist in one-on-one sessions, rather than attend a group Yoga class. Anyone with health concerns, such as many of those mentioned above, should consult a physician before starting any kind of Yoga āsana class. The advice I give in this book is not intended to replace or contradict competent medical care.

How Yoga Became a Healing Tradition

Yoga is a comprehensive system that includes an understanding of optimal health and the conditions that lead to it. Yoga is also a system of interventions (techniques) that can return your body to a state of health. Physical health wasn't the original intent of Yoga; clearer awareness was. But the yogins who experimented with their body/mind to discover how to make it work optimally discovered that a healthy body created a clearer

mind. The writer of the Kula-Arnava-Tantra states (1.22 and 1.24), "For the purpose of attaining knowledge, the virtuous person should preserve the body with effort. Knowledge aims at the Yoga of meditation. He will be liberated quickly. . . . He who does not heal himself from hellish diseases while here on earth, what can he do about diseases when he goes to a place where no remedy exists?"[1]

Many of the practices of Tantra Yoga and Hatha Yoga make up a recipe for super-health. Tantra and Hatha Yoga's body-enhancing methods offer a healing system to those who aren't necessarily spiritual, but who are merely sick or weak and who want to become well. This is known as Yoga therapy, also called restorative Yoga and restorative āsanas.[2] This aspect of Yoga has been developed more fully during the modern evolution of Hatha Yoga, with its emphasis on the physical effects of Yoga āsanas. As a result, many Yoga teachers have acquired specialized training for helping people who might not consider themselves candidates for an ordinary Yoga class.

Practicing Yoga Safely, Whatever Your Condition

Anyone who practices Yoga poses or Yoga breathing practices should abide by the following guidelines. However, a safe style of practice is even more important for someone who is physically challenged.

Practicing Yoga Poses

The key to safe Yoga pose practice is to avoid pain and strain. This means not attempting any exercise that you fear

[1]Feuerstein, *Tantra: The Path of Ecstasy,* 54.
[2]For more information, contact the International Association of Yoga Therapists, P.O. Box 12890, Prescott, AZ 86304, 928-541-0004. E-mail: mail@iayt.org; Website: http://www.iayt.org.

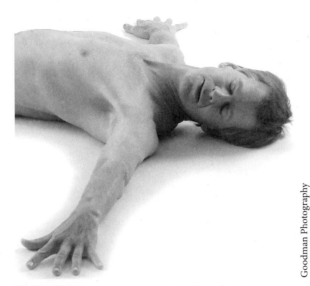

Goodman Photography

PHOTO 7.2   Invent a version of each pose for yourself that works your muscles, but not to the point of strain. Exit a pose when any of your muscles tell you it is time to.

could hurt you, not competing with others, paying close attention to your sensations all the time, being gentle with yourself, and moving slowly.

Further keys to safe Yoga āsana practice are:

Keep breathing with all your movements; don't hold your breath unless it is suggested in the instructions.

Wear enough clothes to stay warm and pick a warm place to practice.

Wait two hours after a meal or, even better, practice in the early morning before breakfast.

Start your practice session with easy poses that will warm up your muscles.

Practicing Yoga Breathing

The main key to safe Yoga breathing practice is the same as for Yoga poses—don't strain. When you are breathing on purpose you should feel comfortable; the effort required should feel slight. If you feel that you continually need to get more air

when you control your breath, if you need to breathe faster and faster, or if you feel agitated, tense, dizzy, or uncomfortable, you should abandon the control for the moment and let your breath be automatic. After your automatic breathing feels truly comfortable again, you may restart the controlled Yoga breath. Don't retry it a third time. Instead, attempt the practice again the next day.

Other keys to safe Yoga breathing practice are:

Always keep some of your attention on relaxing, even while the bulk of your focus is on breathing. Especially relax the muscles that aren't involved in the exercise, like your face, your lower jaw, your arms, and your legs.

Don't attempt Yoga breathing practices that are over your level. A good rule for beginners is to only do practices that incorporate in and out breathing, with no breath holding, or at least only very short pauses after the in or out breath.

Don't compete with other students. Keep your focus within your own body and keep close track of your comfort level.

How to Adapt Yoga Poses and Yoga Breathing to Specific Needs

Adjusting Poses for When You Are Overweight or Out of Shape

Yoga is an excellent exercise if you are overweight, obese, or have not been exercising at all. But you need to adjust your practice somewhat to make it work best for your body.

Refrain from upside-down poses that involve raising most of your

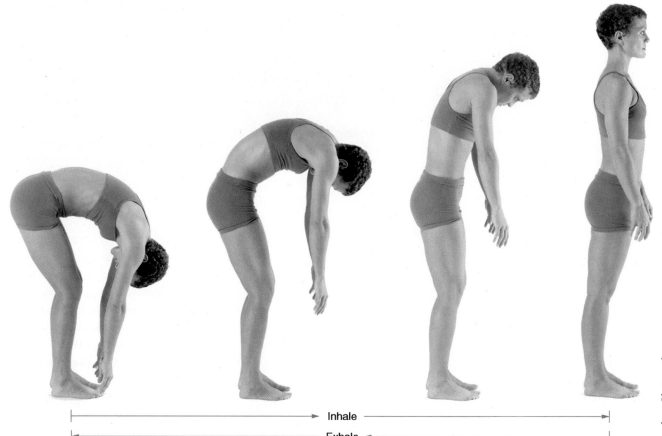

Inhale ⟶

Exhale ⟵

Goodman Photography

PHOTO 7.3 to 7.6

body above your shoulders, principally the shoulder stand, head stand, and plow. These are too hard on your upper back, shoulders, and especially your neck.

Use your muscles. At the same time, avoid straining to achieve a pose or to hold a pose. Invent a version of each pose for yourself that works your muscles, but not to the point of strain. Exit a pose when any of your muscles tell you it is time to. Give yourself permission to do only as many repetitions of a movement as feels good to you, no matter how many repetitions other people in the class are doing. Move slowly. Moving slowly gives you time to sense you body and to stop if you need to. Also, do not jump from one pose to the next, such as to spread your feet when you are standing, as is taught in some traditions. The risks to your joints from jumping aren't worth the benefits of such movements.

Breathe as you move. Don't hold your breath. Generally use inhalations to raise your torso or your limbs, and use exhalations when you lower them. After you have been holding a pose for a while with automatic breathing, prepare to exit the pose by preparing your breath: if you are standing and are bent over, as in the uttan-āsana, exhale, bending your knees a little more, to prepare to rise out of the pose. Then inhale as you rise to an upright standing pose [7.3–7.6].

Focus your imagination on what you can do, not on what you can't do. When you notice you are thinking critical thoughts, such as "my knees are too stiff," bring your focus to your sensations. Your sensations are just as OK as anyone else's sensations. You have a right to feel exactly as you feel. If a sensation seems to repeatedly stimulate a critical, demeaning thought, focus even more intently into the sensation, with curiosity and interest, and keep doing the practice. Many people find that they can quiet their inner critic by persevering with this focus. When bending over while standing, with your feet either together or apart, always bend your knees through the transition positions, as shown in Photos 7.3–7.6. Likewise, when holding partially bent-over poses such as those in which your back is horizontal, keep your knees slightly bent. Again, when you rise out of a bent-over standing pose, bend your knees in the same fashion. Your knee joints are stronger and are therefore safer when they are bent. Bent knees also enable you to use more of your hip-extending muscles to support your torso weight, thereby protecting your lower back. These poses still give you many benefits even though you are not moving into and out of them with straight legs, as others in your class may do.

Adjusting Poses If You Are Experiencing Chronic Pain

When you feel pain you may not feel like exercising. Yet exercise is often an essential component of good pain management. (Consult your doctor, physical therapist, or other healthcare professional to learn if this is true for you.) When exercise is called for, Yoga poses are an excellent way to get it. Even if you find that Yoga movements aren't appropriate for you, you may find that Yoga breathing and relaxation help you manage your pain. A number of studies have shown Yoga to be beneficial in reducing chronic pain and in increasing pain tolerance in people living with chronic pain.[3] Yoga poses relieve pain by releasing tension from your muscles, improving your muscle tone, and releasing brain chemicals such as serotonin that increase your pain threshold.

[3]Kabat-Zinn, "Coping with Chronic Pain" *ReVision*, 66–72.

Adjusting Poses for When You Have Back Pain

Yoga poses can have one of three effects on your back pain: they can help relieve your back pain; they can leave it unchanged; or they can cause you to have more back pain. The difference between these three outcomes is which poses you choose to practice and how you do them. First let's look at how to choose your Yoga poses so you are most likely to reduce your pain and so you can avoid those poses that could aggravate your pain. **Note:** This is a vast subject about which entire books have been written. I will only have space to give you basic guidance here, but I have found that even basic guidelines can be useful both in avoiding back pain and in relieving it.

Poses That Can Reduce Back Pain

Each person's body is different, so you must adjust your practice to your particular situation. When you move slowly and continually monitor your sensations, you can avoid moving in ways that cause you pain.

The series of poses in Photos 7.7 to 7.19 are good for relieving most cases of lower back pain, the most common kind of back pain. These poses are unlikely to aggravate your back, and if practiced regularly, they build strength in your muscles that support your spine, making your back less vulnerable to reinjury. When your back no longer hurts, practice the poses in Photos 7.20 to 7.31 to further develop your spinal-support muscles.

What Causes Back Pain and How Can Yoga Exercise Help It?

Most back pain is caused by tight muscles that are trying to immobilize your spine. These muscles are

Back Pain Relieving Poses

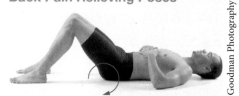

PHOTO 7.7   Pelvic tilt in modified corpse pose a

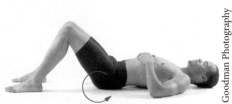

PHOTO 7.8   Pelvic tilt in modified corpse pose b

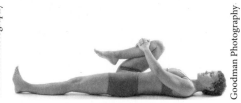

PHOTO 7.9   Modified supine holding big toe pose I

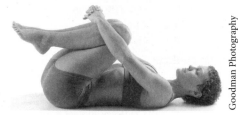

PHOTO 7.10   Modified supine holding big toe pose II

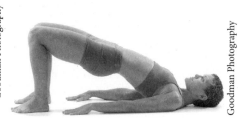

PHOTO 7.11   Bound bridge pose I

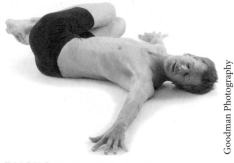

PHOTO 7.12   Belly turning pose

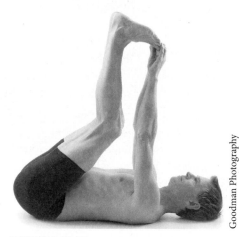

PHOTO 7.13   Upward facing back stretch

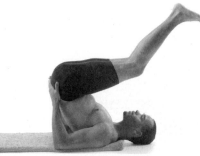

PHOTO 7.14   Incomplete plow pose

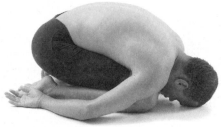

PHOTO 7.15   Child pose a

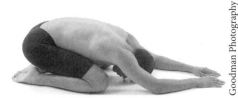

PHOTO 7.16   Child pose b

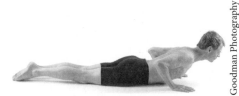

PHOTO 7.17   Cobra pose

reacting to an alarm signal in your central nervous system that says your spine is in danger. The danger to your spine may have been slight, and is probably past, but your muscles don't know this. They still think you are going to fall down, get run into, bend, twist, or lift a heavy weight in such a way that your vertebrae will press together and crush a nerve. These anxious muscles won't let go until they think the coast is clear, that is, until they feel reassured that you won't move in a way that will repeat the dangerous movement.

Your spinal alarm system is more hypersensitive if the muscles that support your spine are weak. This means that ordinary movements are more likely to trigger painful muscle cramps that immobilize parts of your back when your core muscles are insufficiently strong. Yoga āsanas are an excellent way to strengthen these muscles [7.20–7.31]).

Another condition of your spine that makes your alarm system hypersensitive is when your ligaments that hold your vertebrae together are stretched too much. This happens if you repeatedly over-stretch, that is, push past your ouch! point. Some people enjoy this feeling and think they aren't benefiting from Yoga poses unless they feel pain during their practice and feel sore afterward (see Box and Table 7.1).

Back Pain Relieving Poses (Continued)

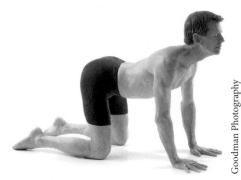

PHOTO 7.18 Tiger breathing a

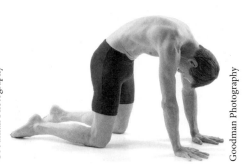

PHOTO 7.19 Tiger breathing b

Core Strength Poses

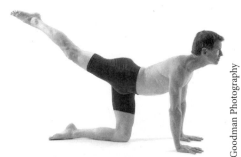

PHOTO 7.20 Cricket action a

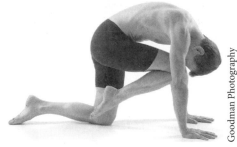

PHOTO 7.21 Cricket action b

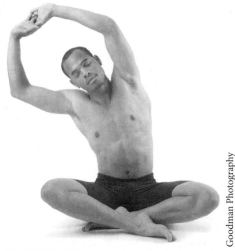

PHOTO 7.22 Sitting side bend

BOX 7.1

Why the "No Pain, No Gain" Approach to Yoga Is Damaging

Your body gives you good feedback about what is healthy for you or damaging for you by giving you feelings of pleasure or pain: pleasure feedback equals healthy and safe, pain feedback equals damaging and dangerous (see Table 7.1). This pleasure-pain equation is especially true for your spine. If you have a tendency to ignore pain and push ahead anyway, you may also do this with your Yoga practice. In a back-bending pose, for example, you may reach the point where you feel intense (but not painful) sensations in your lower back and think, "Not good enough!" Then you may pull or push your body further until it hurts.

The result is this: first, you can stretch your spinal ligaments. Stretched ligaments reduce your spinal column's stability and make your back's nervous system hypervigilant. Ligaments are like straps that hold all your joints together so they work smoothly and precisely. Ligaments also limit the range of arc or rotation that a joint can describe so it stays within the range for which it is designed. Your body tells you when you have reached that limit. It hurts to go past it. If you do this repeatedly, you increase the length of your ligaments so they don't hold your joints together as well. You may think you are "better at Yoga" or that you are improving your flexibility because you can bend further, but you could be making your ligaments too slack or too long, so the affected joint gets a little extra space in it. Picture a ball and socket, like that of your hip joint, in which the ball doesn't fit snugly into the socket. In the case of your spinal vertebrae, extra space on one side can mean too little space on the other side, which can pinch a nerve that passes between the vertebrae. This unstable condition can make your back's nerves sound the alarm more often, causing episodes of back pain. Spinal instability can also make you more prone to intervertebral disc damage.

Second, by stretching to the point of pain you can tear your muscles. In fact, minute muscle tears are the cause of soreness after exercise. A little of this is fine and is a sign that you are challenging your muscles so they will become stronger. A lot of soreness is a sign that you aren't listening to your body enough.

Goodman Photography

Core Strength Poses (Continued)

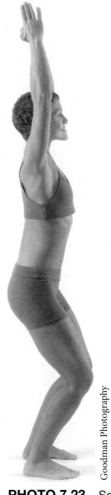

PHOTO 7.23   Squat pose II

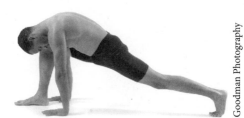

PHOTO 7.24   Warrior pose I a

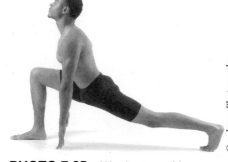

PHOTO 7.25   Warrior pose I b

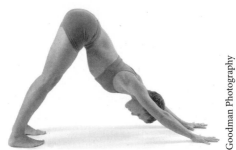

PHOTO 7.26   Downward facing dog

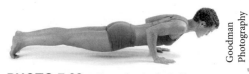

PHOTO 7.28   Four-footed staff pose

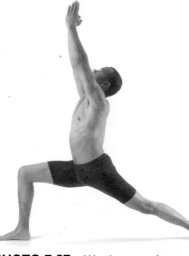

PHOTO 7.27   Warrior pose I

Table 7.1   Safe vs. dangerous ways to do Yoga poses.

Safe, Pleasurable	Dangerous, Uncomfortable/Painful
Lengthening muscles to their full length in such a way that it feels good and doesn't hurt.	Stretching muscles by forcing them past the point of comfort, into pain.
Pulling gently on your ligaments with full joint range of motion, but not to the point of pain.	After reaching a limit to your range of motion in a joint, you push further into discomfort or pain.
Tiring out your muscles gradually, rather than with the first pose you do. Stopping when your muscles become dramatically weaker.	Using maximum effort in your muscles with every pose you do. Continuing to attempt the pose after your muscles have become significantly weaker.
Moving into strange or unfamiliar positions only when they feel safe to you, not when you think you can do it. (To gauge what feels safe, ask your belly what it thinks.)	Attempting a new or exotic pose because the rest of the class is doing it and you think you should be able to do it, even though you feel scared or uneasy about it.
Taking your time, moving slowly. Breathing as you use effort.	Rushing from one pose to another. Holding your breath as you use effort.

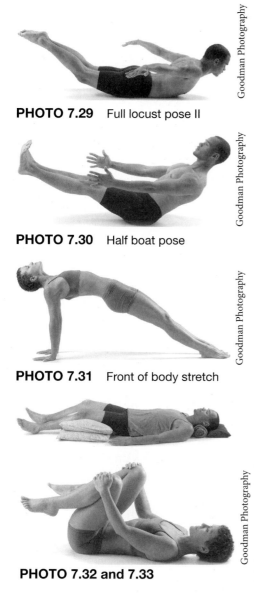

PHOTO 7.29   Full locust pose II

PHOTO 7.30   Half boat pose

PHOTO 7.31   Front of body stretch

PHOTO 7.32 and 7.33

When your nervous system is warning your back muscles to hold on tight, you can reassure your worried spine that the danger is past. You can do this by moving slowly within your comfortable range of motion. Not moving at all will likely prolong your pain; moving too much, so that it hurts, will terrify your nerves all over again, causing your muscles to tighten and immobilize your spine even more. The key is to move slowly while relaxing as much as you can, and only in ways that don't hurt at all. Use the range of motion you have, even though it is very restricted. This varies for each person, so not all the poses shown in Photos 7.7 to 7.19 may work for you. Do whichever ones you can, at least once per day. After each day's āsana practice, rest in the modified corpse pose for back pain, below.

Modified Corpse Pose for Back Pain, Shava-Āsana

Preparation   Get three bed pillows and a rolled-up hand towel. Lie down on your mat.

The Exercise   Place a pillow or two under your knees so that they bend, letting your heels rest on the floor. Tip your pelvis so that your lower back is close to the floor. If you can easily slide your flat hand under your lower back, then move your tailbone toward your feet so that your pelvis tilts your lower back closer to the floor. If your chin juts up and your neck tips back, put a pillow under your head so that your neck is comfortable. With or without a pillow under your head, place the rolled up hand towel under your neck to gently support its arch [7.32]. You may also place your hands on your upper thighs or hips, with your elbows resting on the floor.

Relax your whole body, feeling the places where you press into the floor and relaxing there. Relax your

breathing also. Sense into the place where your back hurts and tell it to relax. Imagine it is becoming warm and soft. Continue this relaxation for five to fifteen minutes. Feel free to fall asleep.

To Finish   Move your pelvis slightly, in micro-movements, gradually increasing the range of your movements, always staying within the range that doesn't hurt at all, or that doesn't increase your pain at all (if your pain is constant). After a minute or two of this, bring your knees slowly up toward your chest and use your hands to draw them closer [7.33]. Hold this for a few minutes, then slowly lower your feet to the floor with your knees bent.

Roll onto your side or stomach before you sit up. Move carefully so as to avoid causing your back to hurt at any point.

Daily Life

When you are going about your daily routines, remain aware of your back so that you can modify your movements and adjust your posture to reduce the pain in your back as much as possible. When you drive your car, you may need to place a small pillow behind your lower back to support it; the same may be true when you're sitting at a desk or in a lecture hall. Especially avoid movements that cause a sharp stabbing pain in your back. This is a time to reassure your spine that you will take care of it; you won't terrify it with dangerous movements. One important way to take care of it is to rest it often, by lying down on your back on the floor or on a bed. This removes the effect of gravity, which compresses your spine when you are upright. Your sensations will tell you how often you need to do this.

As your pain diminishes and you can move more freely, continue to be careful not to startle your back into

Goodman Photography

Tiger breathing

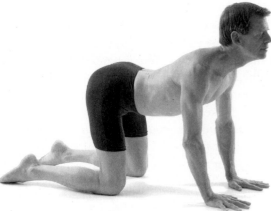

PHOTO 7.34 In   **PHOTO 7.35** Out

Goodman Photography

cramping again. Wait until your back pain is gone (or until your healthcare provider advises you to do so) before returning to a full Yoga pose practice.

Adjusting Yoga Poses for Pregnancy

Yoga poses are a commonly recommended style of exercise for pregnant women. Many Yoga centers and recreation centers offer prenatal Yoga classes. You can continue to take your ordinary Yoga class when you are pregnant as long as you follow a few guidelines, listed below. If you experience complications in your pregnancy, you should only practice Yoga (or engage in other kinds of exercise) if advised to by your healthcare provider. I do not recommend taking up Yoga poses in your second or third trimester if you have never done Yoga before.

Guidelines for Pregnancy

Your ligaments get looser when you are pregnant because you have more of a hormone called relaxin, so it is even more important that you do not over-stretch. (See Box 7.1 "Why the 'No Pain, No Gain,' Approach to Yoga Is Damaging".)

In your first trimester you can do any pose that feels comfortable. Listen to your body even more than you usually do and go for pleasure, avoiding pain and strain.

When your fetus gets larger, sometime early in your second trimester, you will need to avoid lying on your back because of the increasing weight of your baby. You will notice that this position starts to feel uncomfortable. You can either do supine poses in a partial sitting position, leaning back on pillows, or you can do such poses lying on your side. Soon after this you won't be able to lie on your stomach (prone position) either. Consult a prenatal Yoga book for adjustments to prone poses. You will need to be creative to adjust poses this way, but I have seen a number of women in my classes succeed in continuing their Yoga practice into their third trimester.

Avoid upside-down poses after the second trimester, unless you practiced them regularly before you became pregnant and during your early pregnancy. In that case, head stand and shoulder stand can still be done as long as they are comfortable.

If Yoga poses become too uncomfortable in the later stages of pregnancy, stop doing them. Two pairs of poses that you can do up until delivery are shown in Photos 7.34 through 7.37, and are taught on pages 95 to 96. You can also buy a book on prenatal Yoga and supplement your Yoga class practice with a home practice using the poses it recommends.

Yoga breathing and Yoga relaxation are especially useful when you are pregnant, and can be done up until delivery. Of course you can't lie in the corpse pose, but you can do relaxation exercises lying on your side, supported with pillows. Your breathing will become restricted as your growing baby occupies more and more of the space into which your diaphragm used to descend when you inhaled, so your breathing will become more rapid and shallower. But you can still slow it down and deepen it as compared to your autonomic breath, as long as this remains comfortable.

Remember, the Yoga practices you do must feel good. If they don't, stop.

Adjusting Yoga Poses If You Are Menstruating

A common recommendation given by Yoga teachers and in Yoga books is that women who are menstruating should avoid upside-down poses, called inversions, or any pose that places the pelvis above the heart [7.38–7.41]. Many other teachers and books do not give such a warning, and a few *recommend* inversions to women who are menstruating.[4] You can see that this is a controversial subject. I *don't* suggest to my female students that they avoid inversions when they are menstruating, and I know female Yoga experts who give

similar advice.[5] However, as this worry about menses and inversions is such a common one, let's look at some of the theories that support it and some of the evidence against it.

Among those who prohibit inversions for menstruating women, the most common reason given is increased risk of endometriosis. This theory suggests that your menstrual flow can be blocked or reversed by gravity, and that live endometrial cells can be transferred through your fallopian tubes to your abdominal cavity, where they aren't supposed to be, and where they subsequently grow, causing pain, infertility, and other symptoms. I searched the medical literature for studies that supported this theory and found none. The theory of reversed menstrual flow (called "retrograde menstruation"), developed in the 1920s, is called Sampson's Theory. In an article in the *St. Charles Endometriosis Treatment Program Newsletter* (St. Charles Medical Center, Bend, Oregon), David B. Redwine, MD, writes, "If [Sampson] knew what we now know about endometriosis, I'm certain he would not have arrived at the same theory." He further states, "The problem [with the persistence of Sampson's theory in spite of contradictory evidence] lies in the human trait of accepting things from the past without question, and this continues to be our problem today. We need more healthy questioning of authority."[6]

Another theory in Yoga circles for avoiding inversions during

---

[4]Iyengar, *Yoga, the Path to Holistic Health.* Iyengar advises inversions, including the head stand, shoulder stand, and plow, for menstrual pain (p. 359) and for heavy or long periods (pp. 366–367). He also prescribes partial inversions for menstruation in general, to "tone the system." Iyengar specifically prescribes adho-mukha svanasana, prasarita padottanasana, uttanasana, viparita dandasana, and setubandha sarvangasana. These five poses are among twenty he suggests for menstruation (pp. 356–357). Another author, Swami Shivananda Saraswati, recommends shoulder stand for all "menstrual troubles." Saraswati, *Yogic Therapy,* 266.

[5]I have spoken with Barbara Benagh about menstruation and inversions. She writes in an article at yogajournal.com/basics/831, "Since I know of no studies or research that makes a compelling argument to avoid inversions during menstruation, and since menstruation affects each woman differently and can vary from cycle to cycle, I am of the opinion that each woman is responsible for making her own decision."

[6]Redwine, "The Problems With Sampson's Theory: Is it a Theory or an Excuse?" *St. Charles Endometriosis Treatment Program Newsletter.*

Cricket action.

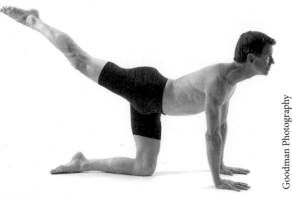

PHOTO 7.36   In

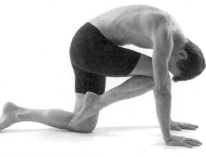

PHOTO 7.37   Out

Poses that raise the pelvis above the heart (inversions).

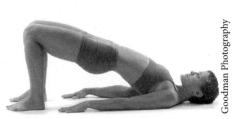

PHOTO 7.38   Bound bridge pose I

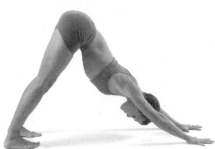

PHOTO 7.39   Downward facing dog

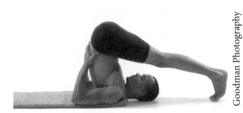

PHOTO 7.40   Plow pose

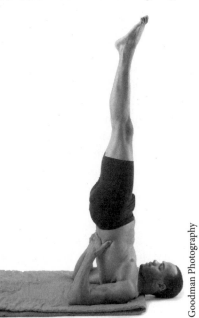

PHOTO 7.41   Shoulder stand

her feeling shaky and disoriented,[7] or resulting in menstrual problems. As with many subtle energy theories in Yoga, this is far from a universal view. As I cite above, Yoga authorities as venerated as B.K.S. Iyengar of Poona, India, recommend inversions as beneficial to a woman who is menstruating.[8] (Elsewhere, however, he warns against inversions during menstruation.[9]

Another theory supporting the inversion prohibition is one espoused by Mary Pullig Schatz, MD.[10] She suggests that the practice of inversions during menses can cause increased bleeding. This bleeding, she writes, results from a state of circulatory congestion caused by gravity pulling on the uterus, which in turn pulls on ligaments that attach it to the pelvis. According to Schatz's theory, this condition squeezes certain blood vessels that pass through these ligaments to the uterus. This leads to temporary congestion of blood in the uterus, which disrupts its normal functioning. I have been unable to

menstruation is that a woman's subtle energy is moving predominantly downward during her period, and that inversions create an opposing upward flow of energy that disturbs her subtle well-being, resulting in

[7]Farhi, *Yoga Mind, Body and Spirit,* 208.

[8]See footnote #4.

[9]Iyengar, *Yoga, the Path to Holistic Health,* 118, 124.

[10]Schatz, *Back Care Basics,* 181–190, 198.

[11]Michael L. Hall, MD, of Denver, Colorado; Daniel C. Austin, MD, of Boulder, Colorado, and Christine Hansen, MD, of Boulder, Colorado.

confirm this theory with three gynecologists with whom I consulted.[11]

The main argument I have been able to find for the inversion prohibition for menstruating women is that many teachers adhere to it. I think it is a theory that warrants re-evaluation. To that end, I suggest that each woman pay close attention to her sensations during her menses, and that she adjust her Yoga practice according to her own insights.

Summary

Yoga poses and Yoga breathing can be adjusted to the needs of nearly anyone who wants to become healthier. We have explored how you can adapt the Yoga teachings to your body, and thereby gain pain relief, increased muscle tone, greater vitality, and increased comfort. Your patience with your body, along with persistent effort, will reward you with new levels of health and wellness.

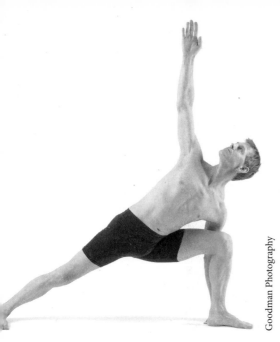

Goodman Photography

8

How to Continue Your Study of Yoga

One person may want to keep feeling the comfort and energy that he experiences after each of his Yoga classes. Another person may discover that her headaches are less frequent when she does Yoga in class regularly. Perhaps she can play soccer better because of Yoga's effects on her muscles and on her stamina. These are all reasons why you might want to continue taking Yoga classes.

Another person may be intrigued by Yoga's history or Yoga's philosophical teachings about the possibilities of contented states of consciousness. He may have had glimpses in class of total relief from his worrisome thoughts.

Another person may discover that she drank less alcohol during her semester of Yoga, or that she stopped smoking. So she wants to continue taking Yoga as an aid to maintaining her good habits.

All of these are reasons I have heard for college students to continue with Yoga (for a few more, see Box 8.1).

Continuing with Yoga usually means finding a teacher and a group of people with whom to practice. It can also mean developing your own practice at home, and finding inspiring books on Yoga to read. You may even feel like becoming a Yoga teacher yourself, which would require that you choose a Yoga teacher training that you could attend. This chapter will help you continue your study and practice of Yoga in all of these ways.

Taking Other Yoga Classes
Choosing a Class

Lots of Yoga classes are available in most cities, but they are not all equally appropriate for you. Here are some of the questions you may wish to ask yourself in order to narrow your search.

Do You Want to Continue to Study in the Same Tradition?

If you want to study in the tradition used in the class you are presently taking, you need to learn something about it from your teacher. Consult the section "Choosing a Yoga Style or Lineage," page 156, and ask your teacher if he or she has studied any of these, or if his or her style is similar to any of these major traditions. Other similarly trained teachers would be good candidates for you to study with. However, you may need to be creative, because not all traditions are taught in

A Few More Reasons College Students Wish to Continue Yoga

From students at Naropa University:

I'm happy to have discovered Yoga because it has changed my life in many positive ways. Although I'm not as disciplined about my practice as I would ideally like to be, I've been consistently doing more and more since the semester began, and I have insights into how wonderful it would be to always start my day with Yoga. I aspire to make it my life practice.

Yoga has helped me to relax more in my day to day life this semester. It has helped me to clean out some of the cobwebs of my mind. I feel I am more aware and in control of my emotions. . . . I was doing great until I started missing class. Our reading assignment said, if you leave the discipline of Yoga after doing it for a while it will lead to bewilderment. It was right. In the time I was gone from class, I began to think too much. I can definitely feel the difference. I finally remembered to breathe yesterday. I also remembered how good it felt when I was in class, how much more relaxed I was and how little things didn't seem to bother me. I want to go back to that.

Standing in alignment (a goal of a certain Yoga pose curriculum) feels more natural and spacious. It is a state of being open and loving: rays of energy flow through me and nothing separates me from that which surrounds me. One night I was leaving school. The weather was warm and breezy, almost tropical for a November night. As I rode my bike down Arapahoe, I felt wonderful. It was not a high feeling exactly; the sensation was more like peaceful soaring. My body was porous, as if I embodied the wind and all its elements. I saw a green traffic light reflect on the side of a truck. This green that I have witnessed thousands of times was more vivid and electric. It was not simply green, it had texture and variety. This lasted for less than a minute, but it was amazing. The wisdom I gained from this experience is that every day is sublime. There is a magic quality to the seemingly mundane. It inspires me to do more work and continue to wake up my mind and body.

every city or town. If you are studying Kripalu Yoga at your university or college, when you go home you may need to try out other kinds of Yoga if there are no Kripalu teachers there. Try classes in several Yoga traditions that sound like they will fit your needs.

Do You Want to Explore Other Styles of Yoga?

Perhaps you'd like to study other aspects of Yoga than those taught in your current class. (See "Major Yoga Traditions in North America," page 156.) Your search will be easier and you will be more likely to find a class

that satisfies your needs if you follow these guidelines:

Be Open-Minded about Unfamiliar Styles and New Teachers   Be patient with teachers who are new to you. Many people find that new teachers or unfamiliar Yoga styles feel off-putting at first. The more you liked your old class, the more likely this is to happen. When attending a new class, do your best to look past the things about it that aren't like your old class, and focus on the aspects of the class or the teacher that you do like. Ask regular students in the class what they like about it and see if these elements are ones that you are looking for, too.

Plan to try at least three different traditions before you decide on one.

Choose a Tradition That Matches What You Want from Yoga   If you want to enhance your athletic ability, choose a tradition that specializes in that benefit. If you want to explore your inner self or your states of consciousness, choose a tradition that contains numerous practices that address this goal. If you want to achieve both of these goals, choose one of the more comprehensive traditions. If you think you may want to study Yoga in depth, to advanced levels, choose a tradition that has depth—in the form of a wide variety of practices that work on many aspects of a person, not just on muscles and joints—and that has beginning to advanced practices.

Choose Your Teacher Wisely   The quality of your teacher is as important to your growth in Yoga as is the tradition you select. Finding a Yoga teacher is like finding a friend. He or she needs to be someone you can relax around and whom you trust. For this reason, when you're pretty sure you know which tradition you want to study, try classes with several instructors of that lineage (if available), and then choose one. Training of Yoga teachers varies widely. Some yoga centers offer quick and superficial weekend-long teacher training sessions and award "certificates" to teach Yoga. In contrast to that, some Yoga centers conduct three-year-long trainings. You can find everything in between, too, with the usual training being two weeks long. This makes the credential "certified Yoga teacher" somewhat unreliable. What to do? Ask questions, and more questions, of your instructors. Ask your instructors who trained them, and how many hours of teacher training

they received. Well-trained teachers are proud of their Yoga education and welcome such questions. If their answers seem evasive or vague, find another teacher.

For comparison purposes, one standard of training that has become widely accepted is The Yoga Alliance's, an organization that "registers" Yoga teachers in the United States (http://www.yogaalliance.org). The Yoga Alliance recognizes three levels of training: a 200-hour level (160 contact hours, about 3 weeks of residential training), a 500-hour level (350 contact hours, about 2 months of residential training) and an "E," or "experienced," level (E-RYT 200s have at least 2 years and 1,000 hours teaching experience. And E-RYT 500s have at least 4 years and 2,000 hours of teaching experience).[1] Teachers who are registered with the Yoga Alliance usually put "RYT," for "Registered Yoga Teacher," after their names, and they may specify their level (200 or 500).[2] But many Yoga teachers haven't registered with the Yoga Alliance, so it is still best to ask a teacher specifically about the hours of training he or she underwent, whether he or she is registered or not. Ask how many hours of teacher training ordinarily qualify one to teach in the particular lineage your teacher uses. However, many lineages don't have such standards, and many teachers obtain their training from a variety of sources; so, the "How were you trained?" question may have a long answer. Be patient, and be persistent.

How to Explore Two or More Traditions   I have known many Yoga

---

[1] Yoga Alliance, 122 W. Lancaster Ave., Suite 204, Reading, PA 19607-1874, 877-964-2255, http://www.yogaalliance.org.

[2] In early 2010, 25,972 Yoga teachers in the USA and Canada were registered with the Yoga Alliance. 1171 schools in the USA and Canada were registered as meeting the Yoga Alliance's minimum standards.

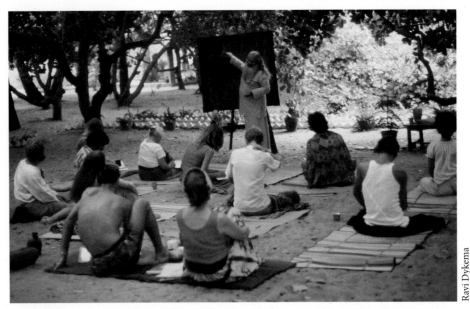

Ravi Dykema

PHOTO 8.1   A class at a Yoga school in India.

students who take classes in two or more traditions. This is frowned on in the Indian Yoga lineages because different Yoga schools often contradict one another, confusing the student and reducing his or her commitment to or faith in the teaching and the teacher. I think studying in several traditions can be useful if you adopt one of them as your main window into Yoga's wisdom, go deeply into that lineage, and use the other(s) as a complementary viewpoint. Another trend is to study Yoga poses for the exercise benefit and to also study meditation from the Buddhist tradition (or some other non-Yoga tradition). As you have learned, Yoga contains a rich meditation curriculum, which combines well with the other phases of Yoga, such as poses and breathing. The problem is that it is not often offered in the centers that offer classes in poses. So if you are interested in Yoga for both exercise and meditation, you may have to find a meditation teacher in your town from a different Yoga lineage, or from outside of the Yoga tradition altogether.

Choosing a Yoga Style or Lineage

Major Yoga Traditions in North America

The following are all traditions that include āsana practice as an essential component.

When a Yoga class is called "Hatha Yoga," as distinct from, say, "Iyengar Yoga," it means it is likely one of the systems that aren't well known by another name or it indicates that the teacher was influenced by numerous Hatha Yoga traditions. It can also mean that the teacher has developed his or her own Yoga system that differs substantially from those he or she studied. All of the lineages and traditions listed (except for Yogananda's) are primarily Hatha Yoga systems, or are distillations of or derived from Hatha Yoga.

Some of these lineages are listed under the name of the guru who is or was the primary source for, or inspiration for, the teachings of that lineage. (Books by many of the teachers listed can be found in the bibliography.)

The Lineage of T. Krishnamacharya (1888–1989)

T. Krishnamacharya's lineage has been the most influential of all the modern Yoga lineages that emphasize āsanas.

The Krishnamacharya \krish-na-ma-char-ya\ Healing and Yoga Foundation (KHYF) Method, Formerly Called Viniyoga   T. K. V. Desikachar is the son of Krishnamacharya and faithfully carries on his father's tradition. He lives in Chennai, India, and travels worldwide. His Yoga is grounded in the Yoga Sūtra of Patanjali, meaning it is comprehensive and involves lifestyle changes as well as many physical practices. It emphasizes customizing Yoga āsanas, breathing techniques, and other practices to the individual. You might choose this tradition if you want to study a comprehensive traditional system of Yoga that includes meditation, or if you are interested in Yoga's healing properties, as this system contains a method of Yoga therapy.

Iyengar Yoga \ay-en-gar yo-ga\ of B. K. S. Iyengar   This is one of the most widely practiced styles of Hatha Yoga, and the system that is becoming the standard for the naming of poses. Iyengar developed his system from his studies with Krishnamacharya, although it differs substantially from the KHYF method. Iyengar Yoga emphasizes precision and alignment in each pose, which is often held for some time. This Yoga includes breath control, meditation, and philosophical studies. Iyengar also developed the use of props such as blocks, blankets, and straps. It is a good system for people looking for a precise physical system of Yoga and is an excellent choice for those wishing to study Yoga therapy. Another advantage to studying this system is that Iyengar Yoga maintains very high standards for teacher education.

Ashtanga Yoga \ahsh-tan-ga yo-ga\ of K. Pattabhi Jois   This is also called "power Yoga," although power Yoga is less strictly choreographed than is Ashtanga Yoga. This is not to be confused with the system similarly named by the author of the Yoga Sūtra, Patanjali (see "Rāja Yoga," page 11, Chapter 1). Jois's system is based on his studies with T. Krishnamacharya, and is energetic and athletic, requiring substantial fitness as a prerequisite. It is āsana-focused and involves a choreographed series of poses done in a continuous flow with breath awareness. The flow is repeated many times, producing sweating and resulting in increases in stamina, strength, elasticity, and ideally, equanimity. In this system the meditative aspects of Yoga are incorporated into the āsana practice. It is a good system for people who want an athletic kind of Yoga.

The Lineage of Swami Kripalvananda (1913–1981)

Kripalu Yoga \kri-pah-loo yo-ga\ Swami Kripalvananda's disciple, Yogi Amrit Desai, began teaching Yoga in the United States in 1960, and later founded Kripalu Center for Yoga and Health in Lenox, Massachusetts. Swami Kripalvananda came to the United States in 1977 and spent the last four years of his life helping to transplant this Yoga tradition in the West. Kripalu Yoga was co-created by a number of people: Yogi Desai, a cadre of American teachers, and a large Yoga community over 20 years.

Yogi Desai has more recently developed Amrit Yoga.

Both Kripalu and Amrit Yoga incorporate breathing, postures, and meditation practiced in tandem with a holistic health lifestyle. This is a Yoga that has retained its traditional emphasis on changing consciousness; it is a good choice if you are looking for a comprehensive system.

The Lineage of Swami Shivananda of Rishikesh, India (1887–1963)

Swami Shivananda is one of the most influential teachers of Hatha Yoga because so many of his disciples came to North America and developed large followings. All of his disciples teach a traditional comprehensive kind of Hatha Yoga in which āsanas are emphasized, but are only a component. These are all good systems to pursue if you wish to undertake a thorough study of Yoga as a means of gaining insight and increased awareness.

Integral Yoga of Swami Satchidananda (1914–2002)

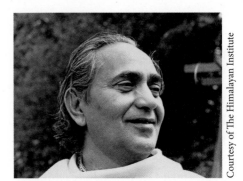

PHOTO 8.2   Swami Rama.

Shivananda Yoga (pronounced shee-va-nan-da yo-ga) of Swami Vishnudevananda (1927–1993)

Hidden Language Yoga of Swami Shivananda Radha (1911–1995)

Hatha Yoga and Swara Yoga (pronounced swah-ra yo-ga) of Swami Satyananda Saraswati (1923–). This system incorporates more elements of Tantra Yoga than do the other Yoga systems developed by Swami Shivananda's disciples, making it the most thorough and complex of this group.

The Lineage of Swami Paramahansa Yogananda (1893–1952)

Yogananda founded the Self Realization Fellowship in 1920 and wrote a classic book, *Autobiography of a Yogi*. He taught Kriya Yoga, which combines devotion, chanting, meditation, and some elements of Hatha Yoga, but not many poses. His successors developed more elaborate āsana systems.

Ananda Yoga \ah-nan-da yo-ga\ of Swami Kriyananda   Ananda Yoga was created by Swami Kriyananda, an American, who was a direct disciple of Paramahansa Yogananda. Ananda Yoga holds closely to Yogananda's teachings and includes a gentle posture (āsana) system that is used as preparation for meditation.

Bikram Yoga \beek-ram yo-ga\ of Bikram Choudhury   Choudhury studied with Yogananda's brother, Bishnu Ghosh. His system is more simplified and standardized than any other Yoga system, and is completely different from Kriya Yoga and Ananda Yoga. Bikram Yoga contains twenty-six poses and two breathing practices, done in a very hot (100° or more) room. The poses are done in the same order and in the same way every time. They require substantial strength and balance, although beginners

may enjoy attempting the poses, too. Bikram Yoga is a good system for people who like heat and want a simple, purely physical kind of exercise that emphasizes strength and elasticity.

The Lineage of Swami Rama (1925–1996)

The Himalayan Institute was founded in 1971 by Swami Rama [8.2], author of the best-selling *Living with the Himalayan Masters* and numerous other titles. It is now headed by Pandit Rajmani Tigunait, Ph.D. The Himalayan Institute's approach to Yoga is rooted in the teachings of ancient India—a heritage preserved in Sanskrit scriptures as well as through an oral tradition. Researchers affiliated with The Himalayan Institute have contributed greatly to our scientific understanding of Yoga's effects. The Institute's Yoga style is comprehensive, classical, and meditatively oriented. The Institute trains and certifies teachers in its method. This is an excellent method to pursue if you are interested in a complex traditional Yoga system and you are interested in Yoga therapy.

Kundalini Yoga \koon-da-li-ni yo-ga\ of Yogi Bhajan   An unusual system compared to other Hatha Yoga systems, Kundalini Yoga combines uniquely executed poses, often requiring intense sustained effort; chanting in the tradition of Sikhism, a religion of North India; and breathing practices. More than any other Yoga system, Kundalini Yoga uses repetition, with a single pose often repeated for five to ten minutes. Kundalini Yoga emphasizes meditation, healing, and devotion. It is a good system for people who want a comprehensive, energetic Yoga system, and for those who are interested in Yoga therapy.

Newer Synthesis Systems

Anusara Yoga \a-nu-sah-ra yo-ga\ of John Friend   This is an Iyengar-influenced (see above) Yoga system that emphasizes bodily alignment and the divinity of one's body and mind, just as they are. It is a comprehensive system that would be a good choice for people who prefer exacting but less competitive styles of Hatha Yoga, blended with meditation.

TriYoga of Kali Ray   TriYoga incorporates "the full range of traditional yoga practices," according to TriYoga literature, and includes an āsana system (TriYoga Flows) and "Prāna Vidya," a combination of breathing practices, concentration techniques, and meditation. This is a good choice if you want to focus on Yoga poses along with meditation in an updated format.

Jivamukti Yoga \jee-va-mook-ti yo-ga\ of David Life and Sharon Gannon   Jivamukti is an athletic, spiritually based system inspired by K. Pattabhi Jois (see above), Sri Brahmananda Sarasvati (formerly Ramamurti Mishra, MD), and others. Choose Jivamukti Yoga if you want challenging poses with a solid grounding in ethics (especially nonviolence and vegetarianism) and classical Yoga goals.

ISHTA Yoga of Alan Finger   ISHTA stands for the "Integrated Science of Hatha, Tantra, and Ayurveda." (Ayurveda is an indigenous Indian medical system.) It incorporates the flowing poses of the Krishnamacharya lineage (see above), the more vigorous flowing poses of Ashtanga yoga (of Pattabhi Jois, see above), and the careful alignment and use of props of Iyengar yoga (see above), as well as various forms of meditation and relaxation. ISHTA Yoga includes the Tantric philosophy that recognizes the perfection in all beings. This is a good choice for those who want a modern āsana-focused Yoga system that is also comprehensive.

White Lotus Yoga of Ganga White and Tracey Rich   This is a nontraditional system that synthesizes many influences, especially the Shivananda lineage and the Krishnamacharya lineage (see above for both). White Lotus Yoga emphasizes awareness, alignment, and breath in the practice of poses. This is a good system for people who want a modern physical Yoga system.

Donna Farhi's Hatha Yoga Method   This method can best be described as embodied spirituality where the emphasis is placed on realization, which is anchored in the body. Although Farhi [8.3] began her studies with Iyengar Yoga, her method reflects a commitment to honor tradition while at the same time recognizing that authentic Yoga is always in a process of evolution and therefore must reflect modalities and practices that are relevant to contemporary life. Farhi's Yoga teaching focuses on universal movement and living principles that can be applied regardless of the style of Yoga being practiced. Although she does not certify teachers, she offers advanced teacher trainings and Yoga intensives worldwide.

Power Yoga of Baron Baptiste   This style of Yoga incorporates a number of elements of traditional Yoga and aims for physical and spiritual change. It is a good choice if you want a challenging āsana-focused Yoga with some meditation and lifestyle recommendations.

A Few Traditions with Smaller Followings

Somatic Yoga of Eleanor Chriswell, EdD   This approach is based on traditional Yoga and modern body-centered psychology. This gentle approach is a good choice if you are interested in the intersection of Yoga and psychology.

Richard Hittleman's Hatha Yoga
Hittleman authored the now-classic Richard Hittleman's Yoga, 28-Day Exercise Plan (Workman, 1975, and still in print!) and starred in the first nationally televised Yoga instruction program, Yoga for Health, which began in 1961. He studied with various teachers in India, including Ramana Maharshi (1880–1950), the great sage of Jnana Yoga (see Chapter 1). Hittleman's books and videos are widely available, and the books have sold over 10 million copies, but few teachers say that they teach his method. I include him here because his influence on modern Yoga in America has been immense.

Gitananda Yoga of Swam Gitananda Giri This is a traditional comprehensive combination of Rāja Yoga and Tantra Yoga, which is also called Rishi Culture Ashtanga Yoga. It was developed by Swami Gitananda Giri (1906–1993). This is the system I study. The main center presenting this lineage in the United States is Naropa University in Boulder, Colorado, where it is offered in a BA program in Traditional Eastern Arts with a Concentration in Yoga Teaching. Gitananda Yoga is an excellent choice if you are interested in an in-depth and complex traditional system of Hatha Yoga and Tantra Yoga. For contact info for many of these lineages and for info on other styles, see Appendix B.

Practicing at Home
Designing Your Own Class or Practice Session

Taking Yoga home means bringing it into your life more potently. Although designing a practice for yourself and finding the discipline to do it regularly is hard for many people, the rewards can be rich and lasting. Imagine that you create for yourself a habit of practicing poses, breathing, and relaxation every day (or nearly every day), and that after you start doing this you feel calmer, your occasional back pain is gone, you have more energy, and you are stronger and better at sports. Let's say that in six months your practice starts to feel routine so you attend a new Yoga class and learn lots of new poses and new ways to do old poses. Now imagine that you continue your Yoga "habit" for twenty more years! Would the effort to get it all started have been worth it?

The best time to start a solo practice of Yoga is when you are taking a class. Your experience in the group with a teacher helps support your discipline at home. So start now! Ask your teacher for suggestions about what to include in your practice, or use the guidelines I give below. In the future, when you aren't in a class, you may find that your home practice gradually disappears. A good way to rejuvenate your Yoga habit is to take another class once or twice a week for six to ten weeks, or longer.

Choose Your Goals

Is your goal fitness, flexibility, relaxation, more energy, improvements in your sleep, pain relief, better concentration, or enlightenment? You can more appropriately select practices from among those you know if you have a goal in mind, such as a feeling or a benefit you want to achieve. If your goal is limberness your body will "ask for" the poses that use your full range of motion in your spine, hips, and shoulders. In other words, you will just feel like doing the poses that produce the effect you want. The key: listen to your body. The more you listen to your body—that is, focus on your sensations—while you practice in class, the more "communicative" it will be when you practice at home.

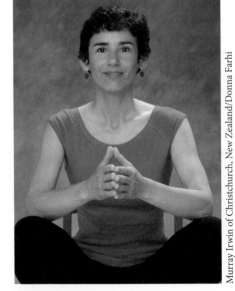

Murray Irwin of Christchurch, New Zealand/Donna Farhi

PHOTO 8.3 Donna Farhi.

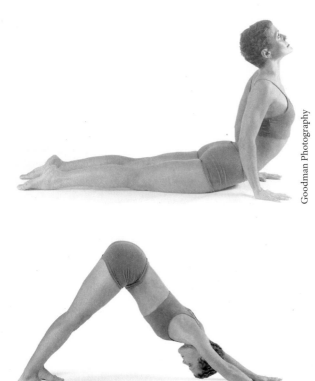

Goodman Photography

PHOTO 8.4   For more energy, pay extra attention to your breath, making sure you exhale completely and inhale deeply.

The following ideas will also help you to design a series of poses, breathing exercises, and relaxation practices.

General Guidelines

Your practice could include all four categories of practice—poses, breath, relaxation, and concentration/meditation—or only one. This will depend on the time you have available and on your goals. I suggest at least three of these categories for most of the goals below: poses, breath, and relaxation, in that order. However, feel free to do poses only, or to change the order—for example, by starting with a breath practice. Many people do only a daily meditation practice and swear by the benefits. The system is very flexible. Experiment with it for yourself.

Fitness

The salutation to the sun (page 121) is a great series to start with. Then choose poses that involve effort, such

as standing and balancing poses, and poses that deepen your breathing. End your poses with tiger breathing, page 87. Follow that with complete breath #2, page 61. End with vital point relaxation, marman kriya, page 117, if you have time.

Limberness

Start with the salutation to the sun, page 112, then choose poses that stretch your muscles and use your full range of motion. Include forward bends (flexion), back bends (extensions), twists, and side bends. Good choices would be poses presented in the "sitting poses" section of Chapter 5, page 87. End with your choice of breath and relaxation practices.

Relaxation

Here are two approaches to reaching a floating, melting, relaxed feeling that lasts for hours: Exercise hard for a while, then do easier movements, and follow that with a long relaxation practice. Or start slowly and easily and continue that way. For this second approach, use poses from the group of floor āsanas. Use a diaphragmatic breath (number 1, 2, or 3), page 52, and any relaxation practice.

Improvements in Your Sleep

Same as for relaxation, but use the first approach: Exercise hard, then relax. The tense and release practice, page 117, is a good choice. Be sure to include a breath, either diaphragmatic breath 1, 2, or 3, page 61, or the complete breath, page 65. Try using these same breaths right before you go to bed, and do the tiger breathing pose, page 87.

More Energy

Choose poses that involve lots of movement and deep breathing. The salutation to the sun, page 121, is a good place to start. Pay extra attention to your breath, making sure you exhale completely and inhale deeply. (Do this only if it feels natural and comfortable.) After the poses, do complete breath #2, page 65. Then do the tense and release relaxation, page 117.

Pain Relief

Choose poses that relax around the area where you feel pain, and that gently move or bring your awareness to the painful area, but without causing any more pain. Some illnesses, such as arthritis, require exercising though the pain, but do this only if your doctor, physical therapist, or Yoga therapist suggests it. Otherwise, use the range of motion and muscle strength that you have without causing any pain, even if this range is quite restricted. Don't exercise torn muscles for a few days after the injury, then do so very gently. Research has shown that meditation helps with chronic pain. Use all of the meditation practices in Chapter 7, and choose one or two to continue with.

Better Concentration

This can be achieved no matter which poses you choose. The key is to concentrate intently the whole time you practice. Focus on your breath continuously, or focus on your sensations without letting your mind wander. This mental effort is like a muscle that can be strengthened. Follow your āsana practice with all four breaths (Chapter 4) in the order given, sitting in the thunderbolt pose or in a chair. End with a meditation practice.

Enlightenment

You have read over and over that the traditional goal of Yoga is enlightenment, which is an effortless abiding in the highest state of awareness that humans can achieve. But before enlightenment we usually experience states I have described as "full awareness, awareness of your true self" and "seeing yourself as you really are." I have also called this goal of Yoga "achieving super-happy and super-clear states of mind." If this is your goal, choose the intermediate goal of better concentration, above. Also establish a meditation practice and commit to it. Work up to thirty to forty-five minutes per day of meditation. If, after trying it for at least two months, you don't like meditation, then do breathing practices followed by relaxation practices for the same amount of time that I recommend for meditation. Also read "Living the Yoga Lifestyle" below. Enlightenment is a lifetime endeavor, so be patient. A continuous relationship with a master teacher of Yoga, who himself or herself has pursued enlightenment, is considered essential within most Yoga lineages.

Living the Yoga Lifestyle

Traditional yogins always made Yoga their lifestyle. All traditional lineages contained guidance about diet, cleanliness, sleep, and many other aspects of living. These old lineages nearly always taught that you needed a guru, or master teacher, to succeed at the Yoga lifestyle. Today, yogins argue about whether that is still a requirement, some suggesting that you can do it on your own, choosing for yourself which Yoga practices and which Yoga lifestyle elements you will adopt, and when. But everyone agrees that you will need teachers along the way; instructions in books will not be enough. Here's a brief summary of eight of the most common lifestyle requirements for yogins:

1. Attempt to live according to the morals and ethics of Yoga, the yama and niyama (see page 25).
2. Pursue cleanliness, that is, wear clean clothes, wash often, brush

your teeth often, and keep your living space clean. Be careful what you put in your body. Also, associate with people who do the same.

3. Live simply. Avoid clutter: in your home, in your schedule, in your relationships.

4. Live in a way that supports optimal health. Make becoming healthy more important than becoming rich or popular.

5. Spend your energy judiciously. Save some of your energy for Yoga practice such as meditation. For some people this may mean one party a week instead of one every night. For others it will mean giving up alcohol.

6. Cultivate calmness and lucidity. This means avoiding too many stimulating distractions in your choice of activities. An example: If you always keep the TV on, try turning it off when you aren't watching it.

7. Eat a healthy diet with lots of fresh vegetables and fruits. Traditional yogins are vegetarians, both for health reasons and to avoid harming animals. (Nonharming is one of the yamas, moral restraints.)

8. Continue to learn more about Yoga through reading and daily practice.

If you are interested in experimenting with the Yoga lifestyle, begin with small steps. Trying to change your habits and lifestyle all at once will stimulate resistance to the changes, creating within you a feeling of being at war with your impulses and desires (e.g., Your mind says, "Don't eat it!" but your body says, "I want it!"). A small step would be to eliminate one junk food snack and instead eat one healthy food each day, rather than vowing that you are going to become a diet purist tomorrow.

Reading about Yoga

Reading about Yoga or reading inspiring words (from any tradition that excites you, whether it is yogic or not) is considered the practice of "self-study," svadhyaya, one of the niyamas of classical Yoga (see page 29).

These are my recommendations for the best books (and a few magazines) about Yoga for college students. Find more information about these books and periodicals in the bibliography.

Instruction in Many Aspects of Hatha Yoga

The Yoga Book—A Practical & Spiritual Guide to Self-Realization, by Stephen Sturgess

Organized according to the eight limbs of Patanjali's Ashtanga Yoga, Sturgess does not emphasize āsanas. He does cover many other parts of Hatha Yoga, however, which are usually left out of Yoga manuals, such as *prānāyāma, mudras* and *bandhas,* cleansing practices, pratyahara, concentration, and meditation.

Refining Your Performance of Āsanas

Yoga Mind, Body and Spirit, by Donna Farhi

This book contains clear writing and excellent detail on how to perform āsanas. Farhi brings your whole body, not only your muscles, into your experience of poses.

Yoga Therapy

Structural Yoga Therapy, by Mukunda Stiles

This book is great for understanding anatomy and for adapting Yoga āsanas to those with special needs.

Anatomy of Hatha Yoga, by H. David Coulter

More technical than Stiles's work, Coulter's is the ultimate reference work on not only āsanas, but also breathing and the nervous system. In spite of its technicality, it is very readable. It requires that you learn anatomical terms, which the book teaches you.

Scholarly Writings on Yoga

The Whole Tradition

To learn about Yoga history, philosophy, and literature, and to put Hatha Yoga (and any other Yoga school) into perspective, I recommend:

The Yoga Tradition, by Georg Feuerstein

Yoga—Immortality and Freedom, by Mircea Eliade

Tantra Yoga

Tantra—The Path of Ecstasy, by Georg Feuerstein

This is a survey of the philosophy and practice of genuine Hindu Tantra. It provides the best background for understanding where Hatha Yoga came from.

Essays and Stories about Using Yoga Every Day

Bringing Yoga to Life, the Everyday Practice of Enlightened Living, by Donna Farhi

This book contains lyrical and insightful essays on how anyone can enrich their life with Yoga principals and practice.

Reference Books on Yoga

The Shambhala Encyclopedia of Yoga, by Georg Feuerstein

The Perennial Dictionary of World Religions, edited by Keith Crim

These are essential reference works for anyone who studies Yoga literature. Feuerstein's work has many more Yoga-related entries, while Crim's includes more detail in its entries.

Biography

Autobiography of a Yogi, by Paramahansa Yogananda

This is the most-read Yoga biography. Yogananda takes us on a fascinating journey to visit countless yogins and saints, and to share his own evolution into a great Yoga guru. Beautifully written.

Yoga Periodicals

Yoga +

This is from the Himalayan Institute, which was founded by Swami Rama. This glossy, well-edited magazine espouses the Yoga of Swami Rama, along with some other traditions. It offers excellent instruction and commentary on traditional Yoga.
Yoga Journal

The largest circulation Yoga magazine in the United States, *Yoga Journal* has helped grow and define Yoga since its founding by the Iyengar-based California Yoga Teachers' Association in 1975. It is now a beautifully produced glossy lifestyle magazine.
The International Journal of Yoga Therapy

This is an annual professional peer-reviewed journal for Yoga teachers and Yoga therapists with an emphasis on research. *Yoga Therapy Today* is a triannual publication with similar topics to the IJYT, including book reviews and articles of general interest to Yoga teachers, Yoga therapists, and healthcare providers. If you are interested in using Yoga practices for specific ailments, these are the best source of instructions. Both publications are essential reading for all Yoga teachers and Yoga therapists.

Correspondence Course in All Aspects of Yoga

Yoga Step-by-Step, a 52-lesson correspondence course by the late Swami Gitananda (see page 47), and now supervised by Meenakshi Devi Bhavanani

For information, write International Centre for Yoga Education and Research (ICYER), 16-A Mettu Street, Chinnamudaliarchavady, Kottakuppam, TN 605 104, India. Telephone: 0413-622902. Web site: http://www.icyer.com.

Training to Become a Yoga Teacher

I can report from experience that teaching Yoga is a rewarding profession. In addition, as with many other skills, teaching dramatically deepens your understanding of the subject. Many good training programs are available in the United States and Canada (see Appendix B). Here are some points to consider if you are interested in undergoing teacher training.

Personal Fulfillment or Professional Skill?

You may want to deepen your own practice of Yoga, but find that advanced practices are only available though teacher trainings. Many people undergo teacher trainings with no intention of teaching. If you want to teach Yoga professionally, I suggest that you choose a program that will help you both deepen your practice and learn how to teach Yoga poses, relaxation exercises, breathing practices, and meditation to others.

The Economics of Teaching Yoga

You earn two rewards from teaching Yoga: satisfaction and money. Your satisfaction comes from doing what you love and helping others. Your pay is similar to that of fitness instructors at recreation centers and fitness clubs. To learn more, talk to several teachers about their pay per class, and do the math. This is an embarrassing question, I know, but if you are considering a career, you need to ask it. Most full-time Yoga instructors work at several different locations each week, and teach between 8 and 14 classes per week.

Some people are happier working for themselves, and you can potentially earn more by running your own classes (rent space, advertise, etc.), if you can attract substantial numbers of students. This means starting a one-person business, which carries risk. If this interests you, I recommend acquiring business skills to augment your training in Yoga teaching skills. The Yoga teachers who make larger incomes, over $50,000 per year, are those who started small and grew gradually, ending up running medium-sized to large Yoga centers. Starting a Yoga center is similar to starting a small business, requiring lots of ambition to succeed and lots of stamina for long hours of work and low (or no) pay at first. It may sound difficult when you are just dreaming about your future, but the rewards of growing a Yoga business are worth the risk and hard work for many people.

Your choice of training program will be influenced by which of the three kinds of yoga teachers listed above you want to become: a teacher at someone else's facility, an organizer of your own classes, or the owner of a Yoga center. If you are unsure, I suggest you choose the most thorough training you can afford.

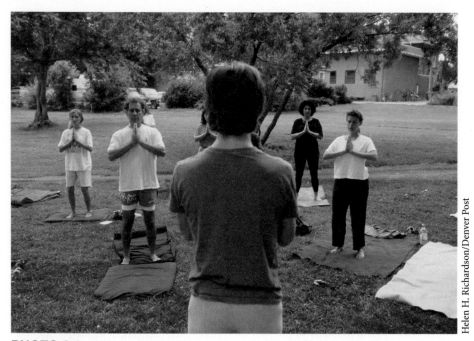

Helen H. Richardson/Denver Post

PHOTO 8.5   Being a Yoga teacher can be a rewarding profession.

How Long Does It Take to Become a Yoga Teacher?

Many residential teacher trainings last two weeks, and grant a "Yoga teaching certificate" upon completion. Some last one month, and a few are much longer. Nonresidential trainings also require varied time commitments. Minimum standards for Yoga teacher education don't exist in the United States, but they do in many European countries. The International Yoga Federation, along with the Latin American Union of Yoga, the Asian Union of Yoga, and the European Yoga Alliance, has developed two levels of training that it considers a minimum for calling oneself a "Yoga teacher." They are a 200-hour standard, which must include at least 160 hours in teacher training classes, and a 500-hour standard, which must include at least 350 hours in teacher training classes. (See "Choose Your Teacher Wisely," page 155.) When you evaluate a training, always assess the number of contact hours the program provides, and then you can calculate how much the organizer charges per contact hour. This way you can realistically compare one program to another, and choose one that offers you the best value, as well as offering you the kind of Yoga experience you want.

How Does One Become a Yoga Therapist?

Most Yoga therapists train first as Yoga teachers, conduct classes for some time, and then study Yoga therapy, which is a specialty offered in only some of the Yoga systems. These systems tend to be the comprehensive ones with elaborate systems of poses, such as the Krishnamacharya method, Iyengar Yoga, Kundalini Yoga, Swama Rama's Yoga, Shivananda Yoga, and Gitananda Yoga. At this writing there are no U.S. minimum standards for Yoga therapists. This profession is still quite young. If you wish to become a Yoga therapist eventually, choose a teacher training in one of the comprehensive systems.

How Does One Choose a Yoga System or Lineage in Which to Become a Teacher?

This is an important decision. Be sure to take many classes from teachers trained in the lineage(s) you are considering before you sign up for the training. If you must find a training near your hometown, you may need to explore one or more unfamiliar systems. See "Major Yoga Traditions in North America," page 156. Also see the contact information for these lineages, and more, in Appendix B, "Resources."

Conclusion

Why continue to study Yoga? A student of mine says it best: "The wisdom I gained from this [Yoga class] is that every day is sublime. There is a magic quality to the seemingly mundane. It inspires me to do more work and continue to wake up my mind and body.

Appendix A

Why Sanskrit?

The vast majority of the literature of Yoga was written in the Sanskrit language. Sanskrit's origins coincide with the Vedas, so the language is at least older than 3000 BCE (see "A Short History of Yoga" in Chapter 1). Sanskrit is called a "dead language" because it has not been used as a primary mode of communication since before the Christian era. It has, however, been in continuous use by hundreds of thousands of Indians, primarily the religious elite, the Brahmins.

Yogins and Hindus hold Sanskrit in high esteem. The sounds that make up its alphabet and the words composed of them are considered more potent than are the sounds and words of other languages. Sanskrit, the word itself, derives from samskrta, meaning "perfected, cultured." Hindus have historically referred to the language as dē vavā ni, meaning "the language of the Gods." (See "Mantra Yoga" in Chapter 1.) Hindus around the world use it for prayer and ceremony. To a lesser extent, yogins do too. For all these reasons, Sanskrit names and terms have followed Yoga poses and Yoga meditation practices to these shores. (See The Perennial Dictionary of World Religions, page 654, for an excellent description of Sanskrit and its literature.)

In the modern world an educated Yoga practitioner is expected to know the most important Sanskrit terms. This will include the names of a few historical figures, terms that describe the theoretical and philosophical concepts central to Yoga, and the names of many poses and a few breathing techniques.

An example of this is the word ā sana. In a beginners' class the teacher will likely use the English equivalent, "pose" or "posture," as in, "This pose is good for your lower back." The teacher of an intermediate class would likely say, "This ā sana helps stretch your hamstrings."

I use the same device, repetition, in this book. Early in the text I introduce the Sanskrit word (in italics) with its English translation, and I may later repeat this dual use of the Sanskrit and English.
As you continue reading, you'll see that eventually I use only the Sanskrit term, because I assume that you have learned it. I only do this with a few of the most important words used in modern Yoga, such as ā sana. I hope that my writing in this way will help you easily learn the essential Sanskrit words you'll need for discussing and reading about Yoga.

Pronunciation

Sanskrit speakers utter sounds that are foreign to those speaking most other languages. An example is a "d" sound made by touching your tongue to the back part of the roof of you mouth. I have not attempted to transliterate this Sanskrit letter (and others like it) into English. I have, however, included a few pronunciation marks to help you pronounce the Sanskrit words more accurately.

A convention of Sanskrit that is easy for us English speakers to master, and that is essential to correct pronunciation, is the Sanskrit vowel sounds. The most common vowel in Sanskrit is the short "a," as in "mantra" (pronounced mahn-trah), which sounds like alone and comply. Second most common is the long "a" as in ā sana, pronounced ah'-sa-na, as in calm and father. (There is no short "a˘" sound in Sanskrit that sounds like bat or carry.) I indicate the long vowel with a line over the letter, as in ā, ē, ī, and ū. The short vowel simply lacks the line. See the pronunciation guide below. (Note that these marks and the terms "long" and "short" mean different things when applied to English.)

The short and long vowel sounds lend accents to syllables in Sanskrit, which otherwise are devoid of accents. So the word ashtanga (ahsh-tan-ga) has no accented syllable, whereas ā sana (ah'-sa-na) does.

Another easily mastered characteristic of Sanskrit is the aspirated consonants. The sound "g," for example, can be pronounced as in "bug" or "gut." Or it can be pronounced while letting more breath out, as in pighair. There is no "th" sound in Sanskrit, as in thin or truth. So "hatha," as in Hatha Yoga, is pronounced hut-ha, as in anthill or hothouse. Another consonant, "bh," used in bhakti (bhuk-tee), is aspirated, as in abhor, while brahmin (brah-min) is not, as in brother.

Vowels

a, as in *a*lone or c*o*mply: m*a*ntra, mahn-trah (power sound)

ā, as in c*a*lm or f*a*ther: ā sana, ah'-sa-na (pose)

i, as in p*i*t or d*i*m: shakti, shuk-tih (energy)

ī, as in *e*qual or b*ee*: nā dī, nah-dee (subtle energy pathways)

u, as in d*u*de or f*oo*d: guru, goo-roo (a spiritual authority)

ū, as in *oo*ze or r*u*le: sū tra, soo'-tra (thread)

Consonants with More Breath (Aspirated)

bh, as in a*bh*or or ri*bh*ouse: *bh*akti, bhuk-tih (devotion)

dh, as in a*dh*ere or roa*dh*og: *dh*ā ranā, dha'-ra-nah' (concentration)

kh, as in pic*kh*andle or buc*kh*orn: du*kh*a, dook-ha (suffering)

th, as in an*th*ill or ho*th*ouse: ha*th*a, hut-ha (forceful)

Other aspirated consonants, connoted by an "h" after the letter, are pronounced in the same way.

Exception: sh is pronounced as in English, as in ship or push. There is an aspirated version of "sh" in Sanskrit, but it, along with a number of other pronunciation details, will have to await a more in-depth study of Sanskrit than we can undertake here.

(Note: When ā sana follows a word ending in a short or long a, such as padma, the combination is pronounced pad-mah-sa-na. This convention occurs throughout Sanskrit pronunciation, e.g. Jī va ā tman becomes jeev-aht-ma.)

Yoga Centers in the United States and Canada

Amrit Yoga Institute

Yogi Amrit Desai (also see "The Lineage of Swami Kripalvananda," page 157)

P.O. Box 5340

Salt Springs, FL 32134

(352) 685-3001

http://www.amrityoga.org

info@amrityoga.org

Style: A traditional comprehensive Hatha Yoga and meditation system.

Services: Classes, seminars, teacher trainings.

Ananda

Swami Kriyananda (Donald Walters)

Also see "The Lineage of Swami Paramahansa Yogananda," page 158

14618 Tyler-Foote Rd.

Nevada City, CA 95959

(530) 478-7560

http://www.ananda.org

sanghainfo@ananda.org

Style: Ananda Yoga is based on Kriya Yoga, the method taught by Paramhansa Yogananda, author of the spiritual classic *Autobiography of a Yogi*. This is a comprehensive traditional yoga system that emphasizes devotion.

Services: Classes, teacher trainings, retreats, community living.

Anusara Yoga

John Friend

9400 Grogans Mill Road, Suite 200

The Woodlands, TX 77380

(888) 398-9642

(281) 367-9763

Fax: (281) 367-2744

http://www.anusara.com

oneyoga@anusara.com

Style: Anusara Yoga is a modern synthesis Hatha Yoga system that emphasizes bodily alignment and the divinity of one's body and mind, just as they are. Founded by John Friend in 1997. Friend studied with many teachers, principally Iyengar, Jois, and Swami Chidvilasananda.

Services: Classes, teacher trainings, workshops.

B.K.S. Iyengar Yoga Institute of San Francisco

2404 27th Ave.

San Francisco, CA 94116

(415) 753-0909

Fax: (415) 753-0913

http://www.iyisf.org

info@iyisf.org

Style: Iyengar Yoga emphasizes alignment and correct execution of poses. It makes use of props and includes a Yoga therapy system called "restorative poses."

Services: Classes, teacher trainings, workshops.

CorePower Yoga

3901 W. 32nd Ave.

Denver, CO 80212

(866) 441-9642

Many locations in CO, CA, MN, IL, and OR

http://www.corepoweryoga.com

Style: The creator of CorePower Yoga, Trevor Tice, does not credit any lineages. His company's website states,

"A truly unique yoga practice based on intuition rather than tradition." Teachers must conform to the limited pre-set choreography. The method is characterized by heated rooms (like Bikram) and a flow of poses (like Jois' Ashtanga), with an emphasis on physical benefits.

Services: Classes, teacher trainings.

Gary Kraftsow American Viniyoga Institute

Gary and Mirka Kraftsow

American Viniyoga Institute, LLC

Oakland, CA

(808) 572-1414

http://www.viniyoga.com

info@viniyoga.com

Style: Viniyoga, a comprehensive, personalized traditional yoga system. Gary Kraftsow studied with T.K.V Desikachar.

Services: Classes, personal sessions, retreats, Yoga therapy and Yoga teacher training programs.

The Hard & Soft Astanga Yoga Institute

Beryl Bender Birch & Thom Birch

P.O. Box 5009

East Hampton, NY 11937

(631) 324-8409

http://www.power-yoga.com

yoga@power-yoga.com

Style: Athletic posture-focused style of Hatha Yoga. The Birchs' āsana practice comes from the Krishnamacharya tradition and includes study of the methods of K. Pattabhi Jois, B.K.S. Iyengar and T.K.V. Desikachar.

Services: Classes, teacher trainings, workshops, vacations.

Himalayan Institute

(Also see "The Lineage of Swami Rama," page 158)
952 Bethany Turnpike
Honesdale, PA 18431

(800) 822-4547

(570) 253-5551

Fax: (570) 253-9078

http://www.himalayaninstitute.org

info@himalayaninstitute.org

Style: Classical, meditatively-oriented Yoga. The Institute offers classes in yoga philosophy and psychology, ayurveda, and integrative medicine. It was founded by Swami Rama of the Himalayas (1925-1996) in 1971, and is headed by Pandit Rajmani Tigunait, Ph.D.

Services: A full service Yoga, healing, and retreat center. The Institute publishes the widely available *Yoga+* magazine.

Integral Yoga, Yogaville, Satchidananda Ashram

(Also see "The Lineage of Swami Shivananda," page 157)

108 Yogaville Way

Buckingham, VA 23921

(434) 969-3121

Fax: (434) 969-1303

http://www.Yogaville.org

arc@iyiza.org

Style: Comprehensive traditional Hatha Yoga. The founder, the late Swami Satchidananda, was a student of Swami Shivananda of Rishikesh.

Services: Classes, teacher trainings, retreats, community

Jivamukti Yoga School

David Life and Sharon Gannon

841 Broadway, 2nd Floor

New York, NY 10003

(212) 353-0214

(800) 295-6814

Fax: (212) 995-1313

http://www.jivamuktiyoga.com

info@jivamuktiyoga.com

Style: Jivamukti is an athletic, spiritually-based system inspired by K Pattabhi Jois, Sri Brahmananda Sarasvati (formerly Ramamurti Mishra, M.D.), and others.

Services: Classes, teacher trainings.

Kripalu

Kripalu Yoga (also see "The Lineage of Swami Kripalvananda," page 157)

P.O. Box 309

Stockbridge, MA 01262

(413) 448-3152

(866) 200-5203

Fax: (413) 448-3384

http://www.kripalu.org

guestservices@kripalu.org

Style: Traditional Hatha Yoga: poses, chanting, breathing and meditation, as well as lifestyle suggestions. This is a gentler kind of Yoga with a traditional emphasis on changing consciousness.

Services: Classes, teacher trainings, retreats, community.

The Movement Center

P.O. Box 13310

Portland, OR 97232

(503) 231-0383

http://www.themovementcenter.com

info@themovementcenter.com

Style: Trika Yoga, an Indian Tantric tradition of Kashmir Shaivism. Trika Yoga teaches one to release tensions and allow one's creative energy to flow. Swami Chetanananda is the spiritual director of the Institute. He is the designated successor of Swami Rudrananda (Rudi), who was a disciple of Bhagavan Nityananda.

Services: Classes, retreats, residential programs.

Naropa University

Bachelor of Arts Degree: Yoga Teacher Training Concentration within the Traditional Eastern Arts Department. Also Certificate Program in Yoga Teacher Training.

2130 Arapahoe Ave.

Boulder, CO 80302

(303) 444-0202

Fax: (303) 444-0410

http://www.naropa.edu

inquiry@naropa.edu

Style: Full-spectrum traditional Hatha Yoga and Tantra Yoga, drawing on the Gitananda, Shivananda and Iyengar lineages. This program was originally developed by Ravi Dykema, this book's author.

Services: Full-time 2 and 4-year B.A. Degree programs, or shorter Certificate Program.

The Pierce Yoga Program

1164 North Highland Avenue, NE

Atlanta, GA 30306

(404) 875-7110

Fax: (404) 875-5054

http://www.pierceyoga.com

info@pierceyoga.com

Style: Viniyoga of T.K.V. Desikachar, son of T. Krishnamacharya.

Services: Classes, workshops, newsletter, special events.

Samata International

Larry Payne, Ph.D.

4150 Tivoli Ave.

Los Angeles, CA 90066

(310) 306-8845

http://www.samata.com

samatayoga@earthlink.net

Style: Dr Payne's style is inspired by his study with T.K.V Desikachar. It is oriented toward the needs of middle-aged and older people.

Services: Classes, retreats, training in Yoga teaching and Yoga therapy.

Sivananda Yoga Vedanta Center

(Also see "The Lineage of Swami Shivananda," page 157)

Yoga Camp Headquarters

673 8th Avenue

Val Morin, Quebec

Canada J0T 2R0

(819) 322-3226 or (800) 263-9642 (Canada)

(800) 783-9642 (USA)

Fax: (819) 322-5876

http://www.sivananda.org/camp

HQ@sivananda.org

Style: Comprehensive Hatha Yoga. Swami Vishnudevananda founded this center. He was a disciple of Swami Shivananda of Rishikesh.

Services: Classes, teacher trainings, retreats, vacations, community living.

Traditional Yoga Studies

Brenda Feuerstein

P.O. Box 661

Eastend, SK, S0N 0T0, Canada

tyslearning@sasktel.net

http://www.traditionalyogastudies.com

Services: Distance-learning courses, Yoga research and resources.

TriYoga®

Kali Ray

P.O. Box 6367

Malibu, CA 90264

(310) 589-0600

Fax: (310) 589-0783

http://www.triyoga.com

info@triyoga.com

Style: TriYoga is a comprehensive Hatha Yoga style, including poses, breath and intention. Kali Ray was initiated as a Swami by H. H. Ganapati Sachidananda of Mysore, India.

Services: Classes, teacher trainings, workshops.

Unity Woods Yoga Center

John Schumacher

4853 Cordell Avenue, Suite PH-9

Bethesda, MD 20814

(301) 656-8992

Fax: (301) 656-7792

http://www.unitywoods.com

uwyc@unitywoods.com

Style: Iyengar Yoga.

Services: Classes, workshops.

White Lotus Foundation

Ganga White and Tracey Rich

2500 San Marcos Pass,

Santa Barbara, CA 93105

(805) 964-1944

Fax: (805) 964-9617

http://www.whitelotus.org

info@whitelotus.org

Style: A modern synthesis-style of Hatha Yoga, with influences of Shivananda Yoga, Iyengar Yoga, and others.

Services: Classes, retreats.

Yasodhara Ashram Yoga Study and Retreat Center

(Also see "The Lineage of Swami Shivananda," page 157)

Box 9

Kootenay Bay, B.C.

V0B 1X0

(800) 661-8711

(250) 227-9224

Fax: (250) 227-9494

http://www.yasodhara.org

yashram@yasodhara.org

Style: Comprehensive traditional Hatha Yoga. Founded by the late Swami Shivananda Radha, who was a disciple of Swami Shivananda of Rishikesh.

Services: Classes, teacher trainings, retreats, community living.

Yoga Works

2215 Main St.

Santa Monica, CA 90405

Many locations in CA and NY

(310) 664-6470

http://www.yogaworks.com

Style: Many styles

Services: Classes, teacher trainings, workshops, retreats.

Yoga Centers Abroad
Bihar School of Yoga

Swami Satyananda Saraswati

Ganga Darshan,

Munger 811201, Bihar, India.

91-(0)-6344-222430

Fax 91-(0)-6344-220169

http://www.yogavision.net

Style: Comprehensive traditional Hatha Yoga
and Tantra Yoga, one of the most complete systems
available. Swami Satyananda
was a disciple of Swami Shivananda of Rishikesh.

Services: Residential full-service Yoga school.

British Wheel of Yoga

25 Jermyn Street

Sleaford

Lincs NG34 7RU

01529 306 851

Fax: 01529 303 233

http://www.bwy.org.uk

office@bwy.org.uk

Style: Many styles. This is a large umbrella organization.

Services: Classes, teacher trainings.

International Centre of Yoga Education and Research (ICYER)

(Also see "Gitananda Yoga," page 160)

16-A Mettu Street

Chinnamudaliarchavady

Kottakuppam, TN 605 104, India

0413-622902

http://www.icyer.com

yoganat2001@yahoo.com

Style: Comprehensive traditional Hatha Yoga, traditional
Ashtanga Yoga, and Tantra Yoga, one of the most
complete systems available. Founded by the late
Swami Gitananda Giri, who was the chief successor
to Swami Kanakananda Brighu (Ram Gopal
Majumdhar).

Services: Teacher trainings, books, *Yoga Life* magazine.

Kaivalyadhama

Lonavla (Dist. Pune)

Maharashtra 410 403, India

(02114) 273039

Fax: (02114) 271983

http://www.kdham.com

kdham@vsnl.com

Style: Comprehensive traditional Hatha Yoga.

Services: Workshops, Yoga research, Yoga therapy,
community living.

Krishnamacharya Yoga Mandiram

T.K.V. Desikachar (also see "The Lineage of
T. Krishnamacharya," page 156)

New No.31 (Old #13) Fourth Cross Street

R K Nagar, Chennai - 600 028, India.

91-44-24937998

Fax: 91-44-24613341

http://kym.org; also, http://www.khyf.net

admin@kym.org

Style: This is the home institute of the
T. Krishnamacharya lineage. Directed by
Krishnamacharya's son, T.K.V. Desikachar.

Services: Classes, teacher trainings, Yoga
therapist trainings, clinic, corporate health programs.

Ramamani Iyengar Memorial Yoga Institute

B.K.S. Iyengar (also see "Iyengar Yoga," page 157)

Contact person: Mr. Pandurang Rao, Secretary

1107 B/1, Hare Krishna Mandir Road, Model Colony,
Shivaji Nagar,

Pune 411 016, Maharashtra, India

91-20-25656134

http://www.bksiyengar.com/modules/Institut/RIMYI/
rimyi.htm

info@bksiyengar.com

Style: Iyengar Yoga.

Services: Classes, teacher trainings.

Yoga Biomedical Trust

31 Dagmar Road

London N22 7RT

020-8245 6420

http://www.yogatherapy.org

enquiries@yogatherapy.org

Style: Many styles.

Services: Classes, teacher trainings, workshops, Yoga
therapy, research, retreats, vacations.

Yoga Institute of Santacruz

Shri Yogendra Marg.

Prabhat Colony

Santacruz (E) Mumbai (Bombay)

400055 India

91-22-26110506

http://www.theyogainstitute.org

yogainstitute@gmail.com

Style: Traditional comprehensive Hatha Yoga. This is the
oldest Yoga center in the world.

Services: Classes, teacher trainings, Yoga programs for
schools, retreats, Yoga therapy, workshops.

Yoga Therapy
Integrative Yoga Therapy

Joseph Le Page

1161 E. Marion Street #179

Shelby, NC 28150

(800) 750-9642

(415) 670-9642

http://www.iytyogatherapy.com

info@iytyogatherapy.com

Style: Kripalu Yoga and other styles.

Services: Teacher trainings, Yoga therapist trainings.

Int'l Assn of Yoga Therapists

John Kepner

P.O. Box 12890

Prescott, AZ 86304

928-541-0004

http://www.iayt.org

mail@iayt.org

Services: Classes, yoga therapist training, continuing
education and conferences.

Rocky Mountain Institute of Yoga and Ayurveda

P.O. Box 1091

Boulder, Colorado 80306

(303) 499-2910

http://www.rmiya.org

info@rmiya.org

Style: Traditional Ashtanga Yoga, Iyengar Yoga, and other
styles. Founded by Saraswati Buhrman, who studied
with Yogi Hari Das in Mount Madonna, California.

Services: Classes, teacher trainings, Yoga
therapy, workshops.

Yoga Therapy Rx at Loyola Marymount University

Larry Payne (also see Samata International under "Yoga
Centers")

One LMU Drive

Los Angeles, CA 90045

(310) 338-2358

http://www.lmu.edu/academics/extension/crs/certificates/
yoga_rx.htm

Style: Inspired by the teachings of
T.K.V. Desikachar.

Services: Certificate programs in Yoga therapy and
integrative medicine.

Yoga Organizations

International Yoga Federation

Federación Internacional de Yoga

Oribe 1398

Fray Bentos, Rio Negro, Uruguay

005982-95357712

http://www.internationalyogafederation.net

fiy@yoganet.org

Services: Providing support, standards and international recognition for the Yoga professional and national Yoga organizations.

Latin American Union of Yoga

Unión Latinoamericana de Yoga

Oribe 1398

Fray Bentos, Rio Negro, Uruguay

005982 95357712

http://www.unionlatinoamericanadeyoga.org

info@unionlatinoamericanadeyoga.org

Services: Organizes annual conferences, publishes the magazine *Yoga Integral*.

The Yoga Alliance (of the USA)

1701 Clarendon Blvd, Suite 110

Arlington, VA 22209

(888) 921-9642

Fax: (571) 482 -3336

info@yogaalliance.org

Services: Yoga Alliance registers Yoga teachers who demonstrate qualifications that meet the Alliance's minimum teaching standards: "200-hour" and "500-hour." Yoga Alliance also registers Yoga teacher training programs. (See "How Long Does it Take...?" page 166.)

Glossary

Advaita-vedānta (ahd-vahy-ta vay-dan´-ta): Non-dual Vedanta. A name for the teachings of the Upanishads. Also called Jnana Yoga, the Yoga of discrimination between the real and the unreal.

Arjuna (ahr-joo-na): The hero of the Bhagavad-Gītā, a warrior-prince of the Pandava clan.

Āsana (ah-sa-na): Pose, or posture. In Yoga's early history it meant "firm seat."

Ashtānga Yoga (ahsh-tan´-ga yo-ga): Ashtānga means "eight limbs," so it is "eight-limbed Yoga." 1. This is the name given by Patanjali in his Yoga Sūtra for the system he outlines. It came to also be called Rāja Yoga, royal Yoga. 2. The Yoga system taught by K. Pattabhi Jois of Mysore, India, sometimes called "power Yoga." Jois's Yoga is known for its repetitively performed choreographed series of poses that cause sweating and develop strength, stamina, and calmness.

Ātman (aht´-mun): The self; also the transcendental self that is one with the absolute (Brahman).

Avatāra (ah-va-tah´-ra): Divine descent, or God-man, such as Krishna, who was an incarnation of the god Vishnu.

Bhagavad-Gītā (bha-ga-vad gee-tah): The oldest Yoga scripture (200–300 BCE), it is the story of Arjuna and Krishna on the battlefield.

bhakti (bhuk-tih): Devotion.

Bhakti Yoga (bhuk-tih yo-ga): The Yoga of love and devotion. It is one of the principal branches of Yoga, and one of the oldest.

Brahman (brah-man): Literally, "vast expanse." The unconditioned reality underlying everything, the fundamental self, the absolute.

brahmin (brah-min): A member of the elite class of Hindu society, often called the "priestly class." One versed in the Vedic lore.

chakra (cha-kra): Literally, "wheel." Subtle energy center, of which there are seven—five situated along the spine and two in the head.

desha (deh-sha): Specific places in one's body.

dhāranā (dha´-ra-nah'): Concentration.

dhyāna (dhy-ah'-na): Meditation, when little effort is involved in holding one's mind steady.

ego: One's "self," apart from other selves. One Sanskrit word for ego is aham-kāra (a-ham kah´-ra) or "I-maker."

eka-agratā (also written ekāgratā, ek-ah'-grah-tah'): One-pointed awareness, or one-pointedness. Another word for concentration (dhārana).

extension: Straightening a joint, creating less of an angle with it, or when you bend your spine back, looking up, while sitting.

five bodies: Pancha-kosha (pan-cha ko-sha), or "five sheaths."

flexion: Creating a sharper angle, such as when you bend your elbow, or when you bend your spine forward while sitting.

guru (goo-roo): Literally, "weighty one." A spiritual authority in Hinduism and Yoga.

Hatha Yoga (hut-ha yo-ga): The Yoga of balanced body energy. Hatha means "forceful," so this is also called "forceful Yoga." In an esoteric translation of "hatha," "ha" equals sun and "tha" (pronounced t-ha) equals moon, which metaphorically refers to the right and left flows of energy united (Yoga) in the human body.

Hinduism (hin-doo-ism): The religion of the majority of the people living in India and originating with the Vedas. Yoga and Hinduism share many of the same sacred writings. Hinduism is a diverse religion with many divisions or sects and a huge variety of beliefs.

īshvara (eesh´-va-ra): Lord.

jīva-ātman (written jīvātman, jee´-vaht-mun): One's individual self; what one means when one says, "I."

jnāna (nyah-nah): Wisdom or discrimination.

Jnāna Yoga (nyah-nah yo-ga): The Yoga of discrimination between the real and the unreal, or the Yoga of wisdom (jnāna). Jnāna Yoga is the teaching contained in the early Upanishads, and it is also called advaita-vedānta (ahd-vahy-ta vey-dan´-ta).

karma (kar-ma): The law of cause and effect expressed by the phrase, "As you sow, so also shall you reap." Our karma, the residue from our actions, from this lifetime and from our previous lifetimes, creates our present circumstances.

Karma Yoga (kar-ma yo-ga): The Yoga of selfless action and love, or service to others without desire for reward.

kīrtan (keer´-tahn): A practice of Bhakti Yoga, it includes singing songs of praise to the divine (also called bhajana).

klesha (klay-sha): "Afflictions" or "causes of affliction." Five are named in the Yoga Sūtra: 1. attachment to things, that is, grasping for pleasure; 2. rejection of things, that is, avoiding pain and displeasure; 3. ignorance (of the true nature of the self); 4. I-am-ness; 5. the desire to live (as an ego that grasps and avoids).

Krishna (krish-na): The God-man written about in the Bhagavad-Gītā. He was considered to be a reincarnation of the god Vishnu.

Kriyā Yoga (kree-yah´ yo-ga): The practice of three of the five niyamas, "disciplines," according to Patanjali in the Yoga Sūtra. The three disciplines are austerity (tapas), self-study (svadhyāya), and devotion to the Lord (ishvara-pranidhāna). Also the Yoga taught by Paramahansa Yogananda (1893–1952), and before him, his guru, Swami Srī Yukteshwar Giri.

kundalinī shakti (koon-da-li-nee´ shak-ti): Literally, "serpent energy."

A powerful energy in one's body, which is aroused from its usual dormant state with the diligent and sustained practice of traditional Tantra Yoga and Hatha Yoga.

lineage: Line of ancestors. A Yoga lineage is the teaching that has been passed on from generation to generation. It is often named after a central teacher in the past.

Mahābhārata (ma-ha'-bha'-ra-ta): A sprawling epic of ancient India that teaches about ethics, religion, philosophy, and culture. The Bhagavad-Gītā is one part of the Mahābhārata.

maithunā (mayt-hu-nah'): Ritual sexual intercourse used in the "left-hand path," vama-marga-tantra (va-ma mahr-ga tahn-trah).

mantra (mun-tra): Potent sounds or invocations, nearly always in the Sanskrit language. Some mantras are sounds alone, not words with meaning, such as the sound "om."

Mantra Yoga (mun-tra yo-ga): The Yoga of potent sound. Mantra Yoga is the oldest branch of Yoga, along with Bhakti Yoga.

meditation: 1. The practice of sitting quietly with your eyes closed or open and focusing your attention on one thing, such as your breath, a sound, or an image (for example, the image of the sun). 2. The culmination of successful concentration, or one-pointed mental focusing. When the object of one's focus fills one's field of awareness and one's attention wanders little from this object, one's state of mind is called "meditation," or dhyāna in Sanskrit. 3. The seventh limb of the eight limbs outlined by Patanjali in the Yoga Sūtra.

moksha (moke-shah): "Freedom," specifically from the rounds of birth, death, and rebirth.

mysticism: The pursuit of direct experience of the self, the divine, or ultimate reality.

nāda (nah'-dah): Sounds.

nādī (nah-dee): Literally, "river." Subtle energy pathways in the body.

niyama (nee-ah-ma): The "self-restraints" of purity, contentment, austerity, self-study, and devotion to the lord.

pancha-kosha (pan-cha ko-sha): "Five sheaths" or five bodies.

parama-ātman (also written paramātman, pah-rum aht'-mun): Literally, "greatest self." One's true self or soul. In Yoga literature this Sanskrit word is often represented by the word "Self," with a capital "S."

paramparā (pa-rum-pa-rah'): Literally, "from one to another." It is a system of oral transmission in which a master of Yoga, a guru, adopts a disciple, a shishya.

parasympathetic nervous system: The nervous system you use when you are calm and unafraid.

Patanjali (pa-tan-ja-li): Lived around 100 to 200 CE and wrote the Yoga Sūtra (literally, Yoga thread).

prakriti (pra-kri-ti): One's living self. Also "nature." A term used in the Yoga Sūtra.

prāna (prah-nah): Breath energy or life force.

prānāyāma (prah-nah-yah-ma): "Life force extension," or more commonly, breath control.

pratyāhāra (pra-tyah'-ha'-ra): Sensory withdrawal.

purusha (poo-roo-sha): One's spiritual essence. The divine dimension separate from nature and ordinary human affairs (prakriti). Used in the Yoga Sūtra.

Rāja Yoga (rah'-ja yo-ga): Royal Yoga, or the Yoga of spiritual kings. This title refers to the Yoga system outlined in the Yoga Sūtra by Patanjali, which is also called Ashtānga Yoga.

sādhana (sah'-dha-na): Program of Yoga practices.

sādhu (sah'-dhoo): Truth-seeker, or monk.

samādhi (sum-ahd'-hi): The state of consciousness that is the goal of Yoga. It is said to be indescribable, beyond conception. When it is described, it is said to be a state of super-consciousness or super-clear awareness. Samādhi is also described as awareness of one's divine nature.

Samhitā (sahm-hee-tah'): Literally, "collection." The word refers to the four Vedas and also to certain scriptural works in the tradition of Vaishnavism.

samskāra (sahm-skah'-rah): Literally, "activators" or habits.

shakti (shak-ti): Energy. Also, when capitalized, a name of a goddess.

shaman: A Siberian (northeastern Russian) word that describes a man, or less often a woman, who changes his or her consciousness so that she or he can see, hear, and touch things that ordinary people can't, in order to help a person or a whole community. Shamanism is the philosophy and practice of shamans.

shat-darshana (shaht dar-sha-na): "Six viewpoints" of orthodox Hinduism, one of which is Yoga. All six offer methods for understanding one's true nature.

shat-karma (shaht kar-mah): Literally, "six acts." Purification and cleansing practices.

shishya (shish-ya): Disciple.

Shiva (shee-va): Literally, "goodness." The god of most yogins, the mythical inventor of Yoga, and one of the two most-worshiped gods in Hinduism. (The other is Vishnu.)

shruti (shroo-ti): Literally, "revelation." The term for the teachings contained in the Vedas and the Upanishads. These teachings are considered to have been given to humans by the divine, through a process called revelation.

siddhi (sid-hee): Literally, "accomplishment" or "attainment." Paranormal abilities or magical powers.

sushumnā nādī (soo-shoom-nah' nah'-dee): Literally, "most gracious channel." The central channel (nādī) of your spine.

sympathetic nervous system: The nervous system you use when you are agitated, angry, or afraid.

Tantra (tahn-trah): Literally, "loom." The numerous sacred writings called by this name. This term also refers to Tantrism, the religious philosophy of these scriptures, and to Tantra Yoga. These writings are part of the sacred teachings within both Hinduism and Buddhism, another religion that originated in Northern India. So you will read about Hindu Tantra and Buddhist Tantra. The latter is also called Vajrayana.

Tantra Yoga (tahn-trah yo-ga): The Yoga of energy control. The Sanskrit word Tantra means to extend or stretch out, meaning that knowledge and understanding are extended by its study.

tapas (tah-pahs): Austerities.

Upanishads (oo-pa-ni-shads): Literally, "to sit down close to one's teacher." This genre of Hindu literature is considered sacred revelation (shruti) that refines but does not contradict the earlier Vedic teachings. The Upanishadic teaching is called Vedanta, meaning "the end of the Vedas." More than 200 Upanishads were written by sages as long ago as 1500 BCE and as recently as the twentieth century CE. Some Upanishads are considered to be the source for Jnana Yoga.

vāma-mārga Tantra (vah´-mah mahr´-gah tahn-trah): "Left-hand path" Tantra. The marginalized and oppressed branch of Tantra Yoga that incorporates forbidden (for orthodox yogins) substances such as meat and wine, and which uses ritual sexual intercourse, maithunā (mayt-hu-nah').

Veda or Vedas (vey-da): The oldest scriptures of Hindusim, called collectively samhitā (sahm-hee-tah'), and considered to be given to humans by the divine. The four are the Rig-Veda, Atharva-Veda, Yajur-Veda, and Sāma-Veda.

Vishnu (vish-noo): Literally, "pervader." Vishnu is one of the two most-worshiped Gods among Hindus. (The other is Shiva.) This god comes to Earth as a living being from time to time, most recently as the humans Rāma and Krishna. Hindu mythology suggests that another incarnation of Vishnu is imminent. Such a person is called an avatāra.

yama (yah-ma): The "moral disciplines" of nonharming, truthfulness, nonstealing, chastity, and nongreediness.

yantra (yahn-trah): Potent symbols used for visualization.

Yoga (yo-ga): (Can be written with a capital "Y" or with a lower case "y.") 1. An exercise system designed to achieve muscle extensibility, muscle strength, and balance, along with physical and mental health. 2. Also the traditional Indian system from which the exercise system, above, was developed. The traditional system includes numerous exercises involving one's breath, muscles, joints, and mind. The goal of traditional Yoga is to achieve the mental state called meditation and eventually spiritual realization. 3. Derives from the root "yuj," to yoke, harness, or join together. So Yoga is commonly translated to mean "union." In many Yoga traditions it means the union of your individual self with your universal self, your jiva-ātman (also written jivatman) with your parama-ātman (also written paramātman).

Yoga Sūtra (yo-ga soo´-tra): Sūtra means thread, and is a condensed style of writing used in ancient India. The Yoga Sūtra is a compilation and reformulation of Yoga by Patanjali. Written around 100 to 200 CE, it presents what became known as "classical Yoga," also called Rāja Yoga or Ashtanga Yoga.

yogi (yo-gi), **yogin** (yo-ghin), **yoginī** (yo-ghin-nee'): A dedicated practitioner of Yoga. In Sanskrit yogin denotes a male practitioner, but in English it means both male and female, and that is how I use the word in this book. Traditionally a female practitioner is called a yoginī and a male can be called either yogin or yogi.

Bibliography

Periodicals

Corliss, Richard. "The Power of Yoga." *Time*, April 2001, 54–63.

Dreyfuss, Ira. "Athletes Say Yoga Stretches Abilities," *Boulder Daily Camera*, March 17, 2003.

Journal of the International Association of Yoga Therapists, published by IAYT, P.O. Box 12890 Prescott AZ 86304, USA.

EnlightenNext published by Moksha Press, P.O. Box 2360, Lenox, MA 01240, USA.

Yoga+, published by the Himalayan International Institute, Rural Route 1, Box 1130, Honesdale, PA 18431, USA.

Yoga Journal, published by Active Interest Media, 2054 University Avenue, Suite 600, Berkeley, CA 94704, USA.

Yoga Life, published by Smt. A. B. Meenakshi Devi Bhavanani, c/o ICYER, 16-A, Mettu Street, Chinnamudaliarchavady, Kottakuppam (Via Pondicherry) 605 104, Tamil Nadu, India.

Books

Aranya, Swami Hariharananda. *Yoga Philosophy of Patañjali*. Calcutta, India: Calcutta University Press, 1981.

Avalon, Arthur (Sir John Woodroffe). *The Serpent Power: The Secrets of Tantric and Shaktic Yoga*. New York: Dover Publications, 1974.

Baptiste, Baron. *Journey into Power*. New York: Simon & Schuster, 2002.

Bernard, Theos. *Hatha Yoga*. London: Grey Arrows, 1968.

Birch, Beryl Bender. *Beyond Power Yoga*. New York: Simon & Schuster, 2000.

Campbell, Joseph. *Myths of Light: Eastern Metaphors of the Eternal*. Novato, CA: New World Library, 2003.

Choudhury, Bikram. *Bikram's Beginning Yoga Class*. New York: Jeremy P. Tarcher/Putnam, 2000.

Coulter, H. David. *Anatomy of Hatha Yoga*. Honesdale, PA: Body and Breath, 2001.

Crim, Keith, ed. *The Perennial Dictionary of World Religions*. New York: Harper San Francisco, 1981.

Daniélou, Alain. *Gods of Love and Ecstasy, the Traditions of Shiva and Dionysus*, translated by K. F. Hurry. Rochester, VT: Inner Traditions International, 1992.

———. *Yoga: Mastering the Secrets of Matter and the Universe*. Rochester, VT: Inner Traditions International, 1990.

Desikachar, T.K.V. *The Heart of Yoga: Developing a Personal Practice*. Rochester, VT: Inner Traditions India, 1987.

Douillard, John. *Perfect Health for Kids*. Berkeley, CA: North Atlantic Books, 2004.

Eliade, Mircea. *A History of Religious Ideas*, vol. 1, translated by Willard R. Trask. Chicago, IL: The University of Chicago Press, 1978.

———. *Patanjali and Yoga*, translated by Charles Lam Markmann. New York: Schocken Books, 1975.

———. *Yoga: Immortality and Freedom*. Princeton, NJ: Princeton University Press, 1969.

Farhi, Donna. *Bringing Yoga to Life, the Everyday Practice of Enlightened Living*. San Francisco, CA: Harper San Francisco, 2003.

———. *Yoga Mind, Body and Spirit*. New York: Henry Holt, 2000.

———. *Teaching Yoga, Exploring the Teacher Student Relationship*. Berkeley, CA: Rodmell Press, 2006

Feuerstein, Georg. *The Shambhala Encyclopedia of Yoga*. Boston: Shambhala Publications, 1997.

———. *The Shambhala Guide to Yoga*. Boston and London: Shambhala Publications, 1996.

———. *Tantra: The Path of Ecstasy*. Boston: Shambhala Publications, 1998.

———. *The Yoga Tradition*. Prescott, AZ: Hohm Press, 1998.

Feuerstein, Georg and Stephan Bodian. *Living Yoga: A Comprehensive Guide for Daily Life*. New York: Jeremy P. Tarcher/Perigee, 1993.

Feuerstein, Georg, Subhash Kak, and David Frawley. *In Search of the Cradle of Civilization: New Light on Ancient India*. Wheaton, IL: Quest, 1995.

Feuerstein, Georg and Larry Payne. *Yoga for Dummies*, 2nd edition. Foster City, CA: IDG, 2010.

Frawley, David. *Tantric Yoga and the Wisdom Goddesses*. Salt Lake City, UT: Passage Press, 1994.

Gannon, Sharon and David Life. *Jivamukti Yoga*. New York: Ballantine, 2002.

Gitananda, Swami and Meenakshi Bhavanani. *Yoga and Sports*. Tamil Nadu, India: Satya Press, 1989.

Hewitt, James. *The Complete Yoga Book: Yoga of Breathing, Yoga of Posture, Yoga of Meditation*. New York: Schocken, 1977.

Holleman, Dona and Orit Sen-Gupta. *Dancing the Body of Light: The Future of Yoga*. Amsterdam, The Netherlands: Pandion Enterprises, 2000.

Iyengar, B.K.S. *Light on Prānāyāma: The Yogic Art of Breathing*. New York: Crossroad, 1985.

———. *Yoga, the Path to Holistic Health*. London: Dorling Kindersly, 2001.

Johari, Harish. *Chakras: Energy Centers of Transformation*. Rochester, VT: Destiny, 1987.

———. *Tools for Tantra*. Rochester, VT: Destiny, 1987.

Judith, Anodea. *Eastern Body Western Mind: Psychology and the Chakra System as a Path to the Self*. Berkeley, CA: Celestial Arts, 1996.

Kabat-Zinn, Jon. "Coping with Chronic Pain: An Interview with Jon Kabat-Zinn." *ReVision* (Spring 1984): 66–72.

Khalsa, Dharma Singh and Cameron Stauth. *Meditation as Medicine: Activate the Power of Your Natural Healing Force*. New York: Fireside, 2001.

Kraftsow, Gary. *Yoga for Wellness: Healing with the Timeless Teachings of Viniyoga*. New York: Penguin Group, 1999.

Kramer, Joel and Diana Alstad. *The Guru Papers: Masks of Authoritarian Power*. Berkeley, CA: North Atlantic Books/Frog Ltd., 1993.

Krishna, Gopi. *Living with Kundalini*. Boston and London: Shambhala, 1993.

Lidell, Lucy. *The Shivananda Companion to Yoga*. New York: Simon and Schuster, 1983.

Lowen, Alexander. *Narcissism: Denial of the True Self*. Basingstoke Hampshire, England: Macmillan, 1985.

Maharshi, Ramana. *Talks with Ramana Maharshi: On Realizing Abiding Peace and Happiness* with a Foreword by Ken Wilber and Introduction by Mathew Greenblatt. Carlsbad, CA: Inner Directions, 2000.

Miller, Jeanine. *The Vedas: Harmony, Meditation and Fulfillment*. London: Rider, 1974.

Mohan, A.G. *Yoga for Body, Breath, and Mind*. Portland, OR: Rudra, 1999.

Mookerjee, Ajit. *Kundalinī: The Arousal of the Inner Energy*. Rochester, VT: Destiny, 1996.

Murphy, Michael. *The Future of the Body: Explorations into the Further Evolution of Human Nature*. Los Angeles, CA: Jeremy P. Tarcher, 1992.

Ornstein, Robert and David Sobel. *Healthy Pleasures*. Reading, MA: Addison Wesley, 1989.

Prabhavananda, Swami and Christopher Isherwood. *How to Know God: The Yoga Aphorisms of Patanjali*. Hollywood, CA: Vedanta, 1981.

————. *Patanjali Yoga Sūtras*. Mylapore, Madras, India: Sri Ramakrishna Math, 1981.

Redwine, David B. "The Problem with Sampson's Theory: Is It a Theory or an Excuse?" *St. Charles Endometriosis Treatment Program Newsletter* (Summer 1995).

Saraswati, Swami Satyananda. *Hatha Yoga Pradipika—The Light on Hatha Yoga*. Bihar, India: Sri G. K. Kejriwal, Bihar School of Yoga, 1985.

————. *Teachings of Swami Satyananda Saraswati*. Munger, Bihar, India: Bihar School of Yoga, 1982.

————. *Yoga from Shore to Shore*. Bihar, India: Sharda Press, 1980.

————. *Yogic Therapy: Yogic Way to Cure Diseases*. Assam, India: Brahmachari Yogeswar Umachal Yogashram, 1969.

Sarley, Dinabandhu and Ila Sarley. *The Essentials of Yoga*. New York: Dell, 1999.

Schatz, Mary Pullig. *Back Care Basics: A Doctor's Gentle Yoga Program for Back and Neck Pain Relief*. Berkeley, CA: Rodmell Press, 1992.

Stiles, Mukunda. *Structural Yoga Therapy*. York Beach, ME: Samuel Wiser, 2000.

Sturgess, Stephen. *The Yoga Book: A Practical & Spiritual Guide to Self-Realization*. London: Watkins, 2002.

Vivekananda, Swami. *Raja-Yoga*. Calcutta, India: Advaita Ashrama, 1978.

White, John. (ed.) *Kundalini, Evolution and Enlightenment*. New York: Paragon House, 1990.

Yogananda, Paramahansa. *Autobiography of a Yogi*. Los Angeles, CA: Self-Realization Fellowship, 2003.

Index